THE
CAUSES
AND
PREVENTION
OF CANCER

THE CAUSES AND PREVENTION OF CANCER

Dr. Frederick B. Levenson

STEIN AND DAY/*Publishers*/New York

First published in 1985
Copyright © 1984 by Frederick B. Levenson
All rights reserved, Stein and Day, Incorporated
Designed by Louis A. Ditizio
Printed in the United States of America
STEIN AND DAY/*Publishers*
Scarborough House
Briarcliff Manor, NY 10510

Library of Congress Cataloging in Publication Data

Levenson, Frederick B.
   The causes and prevention of cancer.

   Bibliography: p.
   1. Cancer—Psychological aspects.   2. Carcinogenesis.
3. Cancer—Prevention.   4. Psychotherapy.   I. Title.
[DNLM: 1. Neoplasms—etiology.   2. Neoplasms—prevention
and control.   QZ 200 L657c]
RC263.L38   1984   616.99′4   84-40248
ISBN 0-8128-2972-7

To my children,
to the future,
and to the woman who gave me both

ACKNOWLEDGMENTS

I wish to express my appreciation to Patricia Day and Sol Stein. The sound of this tree falling in the forest has got to be heard. They have made that possible.

I also wish to express my thanks to my family, particularly my wife, Hilary, who did most of the initial typing while pregnant with our third child. She also served as a constructive critic and supporter of all these ideas.

My students and patients deserve a word of thanks for being as interested and encouraging as they have been.

F. Schachter was one of the most important supporters.

Robert Hogg provided invaluable encouragement throughout.

Finally, I would like to express my appreciation for the wonderful eclectic psychological training I received at the California Graduate Institute and for the education in modern psychoanalysis that the Center for Modern Psychoanalysis provided, which have been the basis for many of the ideas in this book.

CONTENTS

THE CAUSES AND PREVENTION OF CANCER

1

The Beginning of an Answer

IN OUR TIME THE MOMENTUM of cancer research has accelerated. But since much of that research has been conducted, by and large, in a maze, it means that scientists have frequently run into blind alleys and come up against stone walls. One man smokes two packs of cigarettes a day. Another does not smoke. The nonsmoker develops lung cancer. The heavy smoker does not. Statistically, we know that heavy smokers develop more lung cancer than nonsmokers, but that doesn't explain *why some nonsmokers get lung cancer and why some heavy smokers do not.* That's an inconvenient question.

Blacks in Africa do not get skin cancer in any significant numbers, presumably because the pigmentation of their skin protects them from the carcinogenic effects of the sun. *But then why do American blacks get skin cancer?* Another inconvenient question. Turn around in the maze and try another route.

The purpose of this book is to lift the reader—layman and

doctor alike—out of the maze to enable them to see the whole field of cancer problems from a bird's eye view. From that higher perspective, perhaps we can ask ourselves an answerable question: what if a unified theory could integrate all the known facts about cancer and answer all the presently unanswered questions?

What if, based on this theory, workable, reasonable methods of *prevention* were now available to us?

What if, based on this theory, there was available as an adjunct to the medical treatments most common today—surgery, chemotherapy, and radiation—a form of treatment that would increase the probability of survival of anyone already suffering from cancer?

It is the purpose of this book to answer these questions in a manner than will be useful to laymen and physicians, to replace rampant fear with insight and high hope.

A word of caution. When I speak about these subjects to laymen, I try to present the material in as simple a way as is consistent with understanding, without scientific jargon. When I talk to colleagues, I use the language they are accustomed to and refer them to sources both familiar and unfamiliar. In this book, I am trying to talk to both laymen and colleagues at the same time. As for the layman who is reading this book not just for understanding the possible answers to one of the great questions of our time, but who needs the information urgently because he or a loved one or a friend has cancer now and needs to know how and why this new unified theory may help, I suggest that he may want to skip Chapter 4, in which I deal with the question of the genetic or viral causes of cancer; chapter 4 is for the scientists and the scientifically minded.

Chapters 11 and 12 deal with treatment and are therefore directed to the physicians and others who will refer patients for the new adjunct to treatment that is the subject of this book, but there is no harm in patients or friends of patients eavesdropping on what I am saying to the professionals; so I have tried to keep the language in those chapters accessible to everyone.

However, I would like to urge all of my readers to read the book in the order in which the chapters are presented because if you are a layman, and your purpose is practical, you should be familiar with the theory behind the recommended practice for prevention and treatment. And in some respects, many physicians will want to read the book for two reasons: to benefit their patients and to benefit themselves. Doctors get cancer, too. Ironically, oncologists (cancer specialists) have a higher rate of cancer than doctors with other specialties; and since cancer is not catching, the answer to that previously puzzling statistic is also answered by the unified theory.

For many many centuries, physicians have concerned themselves with understanding the functioning of the body and its organs. But the function of one organ has been studied—not by doctors as much as by philosophers—for even longer: the mind. But it is only within the last century and a half that we have begun to study at an accelerated pace the connection between the function and malfunction of the mind and the function and malfunction of the body. The phrase "psychosomatic medicine" has even come into commonplace usage, but in understanding the dramatic association of mind and body we are still infants rubbing our eyes and just beginning to see.

All of us who are parents have seen a young infant, when crying or screaming, splaying out its arms and legs. We usually do not recognize that as a discharge of tension and its consequent irritation. While this assertion may mean nothing to you now, it will mean much when you have finished this book because you will then know the fundamentals for raising a child in a non-carcinogenic human environment and for helping yourself reverse the time bombs that may have been set ticking in your body inadvertently a long time ago.

15

But, in the meantime, when you are considering whether there is any truth to the idea that the baby is getting rid of potentially dangerous irritation by splaying its arms and legs, consider this, too: *the voluntary muscles and fingers and toes are relatively rarely the primary site of cancer because they discharge their irritants in exercise.* The organ systems that cannot discharge irritation are far more vulnerable to cancer. And cancers tend to develop first at the locus of an individual's usual irritation, which is why this book, once it is understood, may be so practical for both prevention and treatment. All that is required of the reader is an open mind looking down on the whole maze so that we can find our way to the central explanation.

What causes cancer, all cancer? The conventional response is that there are many kinds of cancer and, therefore, there may be many causes. *There is no scientific basis for this conclusion.*

Why do some people get cancer and others do not? We spoke of the nonsmoker who develops lung cancer and the heavy smoker who does not. Why are some people more at risk than others? The same question, of course, can be asked about any carcinogen.

For all the millions spent on research, medical science has yet to come up with acceptable answers to these questions. None of the studies help us understand *why* we get cancer.

A carcinogen is any entity that sufficiently irritates the body so as to cause cancer. Carcinogens may be chemical (nicotine), physical (X rays), or emotional (stress). What we have known all along is that irritation leads to cancer. What has not adequately been studied is exactly how irritation leads to cancer. Certainly irritation, both emotional and chemical, is something everyone is exposed to. Why then doesn't everyone develop cancer? Why is it that the elderly and the young are statistically more likely to get cancer? Why do some people get a peptic ulcer in the face of an overabundance of acidity while others develop a malignant stomach tumor? If cancer is genetically caused, why are siblings, even identical twins,* frequently victims of different kinds of cancer?

Why is it that the Surgeon General warns people that cigarette smoking is harmful to their health, but he does not warn them that the type of personality that causes them to smoke two packs a day is perhaps as lethal as tar and nicotine?

The answer to all of these questions lies in *how* cancer is caused rather than in *what* causes cancer.

We come to a curious phenomenon. Though, as I have said, our century has given special credence to the idea that the mind can influence the welfare of the body, the sophisticated cancer reseachers, their eyes glued to their microscopes in the pursuit of answers, have failed to look up long enough to study the behavior of their patients, not when they are smoking or breathing polluted air, but the manner in which they relate to other human beings. One doesn't need a microscope to study human interaction, only a willingness to use one's eyes and ears and intelligence to observe, listen, and compare. If one does, what one learns can be startling.

Because psychological factors have been given only slight acknowledgment by cancer researchers, the complex biological aspects of cancer have not been integrated with the psychological aspects. Yet this integration can provide the answer to all of the questions asked above.

One medical journal editor who read my first articles from which this book evolved had cancer at the time. He had undergone three operations, radiology, and chemotherapy. In our telephone conversations, he made it clear, indirectly, that he was waiting to die.

I asked him if he had ever considered dealing with the emotional aspects of his disorder.

*Green, W., and Swisher, S., 1969.

He replied that his oncologist (a cancer specialist) had told him that he had been given the most potent forms of treatment. To give him any more would result in certain death. When he had asked the doctor if there was anything at all that could be done, the doctor had said there was not.

The editor told me all this because he had read my papers. He said that he fit the description of the cancerous personality very closely and that the background that I described as precancerous coincided with his own experience. He also knew of studies with mice and rats that demonstrated that stress was somehow involved with cancer.

But when I asked him again if he would be willing to investigate the emotional aspects of his illness, he replied that he was so busy with his work and family that psychological treatment would be far too inconvenient.

I asked him if my articles had made any sense to him. He repeated that he felt that they were vitally important. So I asked why he would not follow the recommendations in them. He ignored the question. It was hard to believe, but this man was telling me that he would rather die than deal with the feelings connected with his cancer. He did not want to allow them into his consciousness. It took several months of repeated failure with initial contacts with cancer patients for me to come to understand this. I will explain it later, but for now this episode can be viewed as testimony to some people's need to deny the information in this book.

As I have said, it has been known for a long time that irritation, both chemical and emotional, causes cancer. Knowing this, it is horribly frightening to recognize that the chemical environment we live in is an environment we have almost no control over. It is equally as frightening to recognize that one's own personality and psychological defenses can be even more potent carcinogens than chemicals are.

There are many different types of cancer. Some, such as

malignant tumors, initially attack in localized areas; and some, such as lymphomas, are pervasive. Some, such as leukemia, seem to target specific age populations (the young and the very old); and others, such as testicular or cervical cancer, are related to gender. How can we make any generalization about all these different types of cancer?

If a disorder is to be considered cancer, it must have two characteristic symptoms: *rapid* and apparently *random* reproduction of cells. Medical science still has not been able to tell us what agent or mechanism actually sets up this complex chain of events. We can only deduce the nature of the mechanism by its effects.

Cancer is not directly observable; only its effects are. We can study tumors or leukemia, but we don't have a clear idea of their causes. However, some very revealing information is available as to which people are more likely to develop cancer.

If you are a divorced female living in the United States or England, your chances of suffering from breast or cervical cancer is significantly higher than if you are married or than if you have never been married (up to age 40 or so). If you are a widow, the risks of cancer are even higher than if you are divorced. In Australia it was discovered that loss of a spouse causes lowered immunity to infection.*

Charles Weinstock at the Albert Einstein College of Medicine found another disconcerting fact. If an individual suffered from extensive emotional trauma (such as the loss of a mother) during the first seven years of life and, then, also lost a satisfying relationship during young adulthood, cancer followed within six months to eight years. Weinstock observed that these people also

---

*MacKintosh, S., and Bacon, C. L., 1952; Holmes, T. H., and Madusa, M., 1973; Klopfer, B., 1957; Bartrop, R. W. et al., 1977; and again in a more elaborate study done in the United States in 1983, Dr. Steven Schleifer et al. demonstrated a definite suppression of lymphocyte stimulation following bereavement.

had an inability to relate adequately to others. The latter observation can be considered a subjective one, but keep in mind that the inability to relate is something we all can judge fairly accurately in our friends and acquaintances.

What is more significant is that these people breathe the same air, drink the same fluids, eat the same foods, and are exposed to the same viruses as the rest of us. Why do they run a higher risk of cancer?

The immune system can be less effective in an individual suffering from extreme stress or anxiety. But are we then to believe that married women do not have extremes of stress and anxiety? Married women do get breast and cervical cancer. But if a woman is married and then is unmarried, the odds increase. (I do believe that some marriages are carcinogenic, and I will explain how in a subsequent chapter.)

One can argue that statistics can be found to prove any point, but the hard facts presented here are the kinds we try to ignore because they indicate that we may have some degree of control over the disorder we call cancer. They also indicate that something other than viruses or heredity or external carcinogens is operating. They indicate that something clearly psychological in nature, based on life events, is contributing.

According to Dr. C. J. Johnson, a study was done some time ago of a Mormon community in smog-ridden southern California. Oddly enough, the study showed that this group of people, residing in a carcinogenic greenhouse, was not developing cancer at the rate everyone else was.

The first attack on the results of the study suggested that the researchers had deliberately misrepresented the information by not taking into account the fact that Mormons do not smoke or drink. But further examination showed that the Mormons in southern California do not get any kind of cancer, even those unrelated to environmental pollution, smoking, or drinking, at the "normal rate"; however, the reasons for this were not pursued.

Recently the effects of nuclear testing fallout were studied in Utah by C. J. Johnson. The Mormons again had a significantly lower rate of cancer, and once again, the experts claimed that it was because the Mormons do not smoke or drink.

Mormons in southern California, Utah, or anywhere else are all taught the same things. The most important is that life should be managed through principles of moderation. Perhaps even more important, Mormons belong to someone or something other than themselves. Part of their process of reaching adulthood includes fulfilling missions of giving. And the fact is that they are relatively immune as a group in the midst of a carcinogenic hotbed.*

American Blacks provide more support for the psychosomatic nature of cancer. Albert Schweitzer, when asked if he encountered cancer among his native patients in Africa, replied that he had never seen a case until other white men arrived. Schweitzer made it clear, however, that he was not saying that there was no cancer among his contemporary African Blacks. He was merely saying that with the other diseases he had encountered, he had never seen cancer prior to the arrival of the influence of "civilization."

Apparently this would indicate the lack of a hereditary tendency to cancer. American Blacks, however, suffer from a significantly higher rate of skin cancer than other dark-skinned peoples. Why? Could it be that being black in the United States certainly attaches great psychological significance to your skin?

We know that certain groups have occupational hazards involving cancer. City cab drivers used to get skin cancer on the left arm, which was the one held out in the sun to bake during the

*Spicer, J., and Gustavus, S., 1974; Lyon, J., 1977; and a conversation with Dr. C. J. Johnson, 1984.

summer months. Chimney sweeps used to get skin cancer to an alarming degree. That was before the turn of the century when frequent bathing and the use of soap were uncommon. In England, where the sweeps were lowered into chimneys, skin cancer of the scrotum was common. The harness with which they were lowered down the chimney undoubtedly caused additional irritation to this region of the body; the soot and grime were bad enough, but the harness ground these carcinogens into the scrotum.

The risks are high for anyone working in an asbestos factory. They are even higher for anyone employed in a high-risk job prior to working in an asbestos factory. But some, perhaps many, of these people almost defiantly do not get cancer. Heredity, virology, and present carcinogen theory do not adequately explain these issues of who does, and who does not, wind up with cancer.

The white mice study of the Pacific Northwest Research Foundation in Seattle is frequently used by professionals to show the significance of stress in the development of cancer.* A highly cancer-prone strain of mice was studied. In the laboratory, these mice developed tumors within eight to eighteen months after birth in over 50 percent of the cases. But when the mice were raised in soundproof and protected areas, away from the stimulation of the noises and lights of a laboratory, only 7 percent developed cancer. If the animals were then made to feel greater stress through manipulation, the original incidence of cancer was repeated.

At Stanford Medical School, a study of virus-connected tumors in mice revealed that the tumor size increased if an electric shock was applied to induce stress.

These studies raise the same questions that are raised with external carcinogens. If stress is the ultimate emotional carcino-

*Riley, B., 1975.

gen, then most people living in the United States should be cancerous.

In New York, Los Angeles, Chicago, Denver, Atlanta, or any other large city, noise pollution, traffic, job pressure, and the need to win create enough stress to kill any white mouse. If it were only a matter of chemical carcinogens interacting with emotional stress, we should all have died by no later than 1970.

Looking for a unified explanation of the cause of cancer is like going down the corridor of a maze and being blocked and trying another avenue and being blocked and trying another avenue. But if the maze is looked at from above, starting the observation at the destination, you will soon find yourself able to see the one path that goes through it.

The destination that we have all presumably been hoping for in our research is a theory that will explain not only what we have already learned but all of the puzzling aspects of the maze that are as yet unexplained. In the pursuit of an understanding of cancer, many good men and serious scientists have ended up in blind alleys because they were not working from the possibility of a unified theory.

What I will do is tell you how *all* cancers can be explained. The theory I will present will offer an explanation as to what must happen to make an individual vulnerable to all these toxic influences, how cancer spreads or metastasizes, why some cancers are pervasive and some initially localized, and, most important, I will offer some ideas that I sincerely hope will assist in preventing and curing the disorder.

2

The Beginnings
of Cancer

IN SEARCHING FOR THE CAUSE of a disease, the medical profession, ever since Pasteur, has been conditioned to look for the germ, the virus, the thing. Thus, even though there is considerable evidence that certain personality types are more prone to heart attacks than others, cholesterol and tobacco remain the experts' hands-down favorite causes.

Psychological studies have been even more completely ignored by cancer researchers. Science continues to search for a simple and direct explanation for cancer while ignoring the complexity of the interaction of psychology and biology.

Certainly everyone would be delighted if an effective anti-cancer vaccine could be found, but we do not appear to be anywhere near this; and it may, in fact, be impossible. To find out why requires a serious study of the psychology of cancer.

Psychologically, cancer may be viewed as the ultimate primitive psychosomatic representation of an extreme separation of the self-contained positive and negative forces motivating our lives. It is a resistance to the integration of the basic biologically determined drives of aggression and libido (destructive forces and constructive forces). Cancer is blatantly a narcissistic dysfunction (a self-contained problem), which is evidence of the conflict of these most primitive drives. It is an attack upon the self in which the forces of life are overwhelmed by the person's unconscious self-destructive needs. Cancer is a clash of the forces that Freud and other early psychoanalysts first recognized as innate drives. Most important, cancer can be viewed as the bodily expression of a person's inability to cope with internal or external stimuli. Cancer may be considered to be the accumulation of irritation that triggers a learned bodily defense. This conditioning to irritation may be very specific (a tumor) or pervasive throughout the body (lymphoma or leukemia).

Physical and chemical irritants coming from the outside—caused by air pollution, X rays, Agent Orange, cigarette smoke, to give just a few examples—are external (exogenous) carcinogens. The chemicals arising from within the body that cause irritation to the cells are internal (endogenous) carcinogens. These are far more potentially damaging. They are produced from the body's own defensive structure, and their immediate purpose, in limited dosage and duration, is to ward off irritation. But if the reaction is too strong or prolonged, they cause it.

Adrenaline (epinephrine) is an extremely potent drug. When administered by medical professionals in a hospital, the metering out of the drug is carefully monitored, and an antiadrenaline antidote is always immediately at hand. If you have been conditioned into a state of chronic anxiety and your body is almost always poised for fight or flight, your adrenal glands are working overtime to maintain an excess of this potent drug. Worst of all is the direct access the drug has to many different organ systems and their cells. The cells are confronted with this irritant continuously and directly. This can cause the production of still other irritants.

If you have been conditioned to direct your rage at your upper digestive tract, excess gastric juices will be secreted. Hydrochloric acid will be the primary internal carcinogen. You will be literally eating up your own stomach lining.

Against external carcinogens, we at least have the protection of the skin, nasal hairs, and the ability of the digestive tract not to assimilate some irritants into the bloodstream. We also have an immune system to form antibodies, antigens, benign encapsulating cysts, white blood cells, and so forth. But there are no natural effective screening methods to prevent direct access to the cells by the internal carcinogens.

The effects of smoking and drinking provide examples of the interaction of external and internal carcinogens. If an individual needs to be soothed emotionally by using either of these drugs to excess, he is most likely attempting to contain feelings that are capable of overproducing internal carcinogens.

Kurt is an exceedingly hardworking owner of a small, successful business. His work is seasonal, and his increase in smoking is also seasonal. Kurt made this observation himself:

> When business is busy like this, I smoke maybe two or three packs a day. In the off-season I can hold it down to maybe one or one and a half packs. But then I just sit around and always worry about how the business will survive until the next busy season. I mean it always has survived. I've been doing it for almost twenty years, and by now you would think I'd know and not worry so much. The really crazy part is that when the busy season comes, I have to worry more. I have to worry about the crumbs I hire quitting on me. Then I have to worry about whether enough work is coming in. So I guess it's a never-ending battle of anxiety. By now you'd think I would have learned that this business is a survivor. The question is whether I'm a survivor, too. Sometimes I think I could drop dead from all this aggravation. My wife and kids keep asking me to quit smoking. What they don't know is how much more I smoke than they think. Once in a while I even

have to take a valium to settle down, when the cigarettes aren't enough. If I gave up cigarettes now, you'd have to cart me off to the funny farm. I hate to admit it, but I really need them!

Kurt is a perfect example of a high-risk individual for cancer. Not only is he a heavy smoker, but he is also a heavy generator of internal carcinogens. This interaction of carcinogens from the outside and carcinogens from the inside can cause an explosion. The explosion is cancer.

But paradoxically alcohol and tobacco can also serve as suppressors of the production of internal carcinogens. This should certainly be taken into account by a physician and concerned family members before pressuring an individual to stop their use. Internal carcinogens may be far more damaging than external ones. The internal carcinogens must be dealt with first. If the external carcinogen is removed too soon, it is possible to cause greater damage through the body's reaction to the unchecked feelings released.

This should not be interpreted as an excuse for anyone to continue smoking or excessive drinking. It is only to point out that drug abuse is a symptom of deeper-rooted problems, and the superficial and premature removal of a symptom or defense can have serious emotional consequences.

Cancer patients frequently have a history of their psychology attacking their biology. To understand this, we must start at the beginning—the point at which internal and external influences cannot be separated. It is at this point that they have the greatest potential for interaction. The beginning is really the beginning: pregnancy and infancy.

We have only recently begun attempting to investigate seriously the influences to which the fetus is exposed. In the last ten or twenty years, we have probably learned more about its vulnerability than throughout all of mankind's previous history. We have a much better understanding of genetics, and we are learning more and more about the influence of environment on the fetus. We know that certain drugs taken, or certain illnesses occurring, in the first trimester can result in serious deformity of the fetus. We know that women who smoke during pregnancy give birth to below-average-weight babies, who are also more likely to suffer from respiratory problems early in life. Alcohol abuse may cause retardation.

But we are just beginning to explore scientifically the emotional influences upon the process of pregnancy. We know that the fetus is likely to move less in the second and third trimester when the mother is listening to soothing music.

We also know that the mother is going to produce internal carcinogens in the course of pregnancy. No woman can go through an entire pregnancy without periodic elevation of such chemical irritants. And these chemicals can cross the placental barriers. Why then are not all babies born with some manifestation of suffering?

As a point of interest, almost no one is born with cancer. If it were hereditary this would not be the case. The baby is protected from cancer and other serious damage by a threefold system of defense.

1. The baby can move and through the movement of the voluntary musculature can dissipate irritation.

2. The fetus's own systems for the production of internal carcinogens are still developing. They cannot add substantially to the irritants the mother provides. The nervous system also is not fully developed in terms of its insulation. Discomfort and pain may be less severely experienced.

3. The mother and developing baby are a psychological unit. They are one. Expectant mothers frequently enjoy the sensation of life and can sooth and comfort the fetus through words and by touching their abdomens. This identification and fusion with the fetus is highly protective. It is the most important factor in the protection of the unborn. The mother's defenses, both physically

and emotionally, serve to absorb the fetus's irritations. This phenomenon will be explained later. First, we must take into account some additional issues of human development.

Assuming a healthy baby is the outcome of fertilization of the ovum and a successful pregnancy, what can we say to describe this vulnerable little creature? One word seems to sum it all up: hypersensitivity. The baby, as LeBoyer and others have observed, is a bundle of rawness. A comforting blanket may feel like sandpaper to this skin that has just emerged from months of soothing suspension in the amniotic fluid. Eyes that have never seen light are suddenly overstimulated by even the deliberately dull lighting of an aware hospital's delivery room. Ears that have heard only the softened and muffled noises passed through the mother's tissues and the amniotic fluid suddenly are subjected to the powerful stimulation of even soft voices and perhaps loud medical procedures. Smell and taste have their first opportunity to begin the long process of learning to discriminate.

I have always been amazed by how powerfully sleeping newborns react to smells. The irritating molecules actually seem to cause pain. The body twists and the face contorts in response to pungent odors. Tastes appear to evoke similar responses. Vitamins or iron supplements, perhaps the two most frequently administered medications, cause a sudden recoiling, a contortion of the face, and perhaps even tears. I have observed newborns being exposed to overstimulation of their senses while they were asleep. The reactions were similar to the alert-and-awake state. Physical stimulation of touch, sight, or hearing appeared to elicit less intense reactions. Chemical stimulation appeared to be the most irritating. These chemical reactions are, in my opinion, more potent and more primitive. Lower animal forms continue to rely upon them throughout life. The human animal at birth appears to be hypersensitive to them. The use of "smelling salts" to revive an adult who has fainted clearly demonstrates that the "chemical senses" of taste and smell are more potent than the physical senses of touch, sight, and hearing.

At birth, the baby is immediately introduced to external and internal stimulation that is more than he can tolerate. During the first several months of life, he can defend against such stimulation by withdrawing into sleep or through movement of his voluntary muscles. At this point of human development, the person is at the epitome of narcissism (self-containment). The baby does not have an ability to separate or differentiate between the environment, the people in it, and himself. The baby's cognitive or thought processes are nowhere near that of the adult. Obviously, we do not know what babies may be capable of thinking, but it appears that everything that stimulates, either from the inside out or the outside in is immediately transposed into sensory-motor reactions. The baby feels, and the feelings are immediately transposed into bodily experience. The baby does not have the psychological defenses of an adult or even a child at later stages. Hunger is reacted to with extreme irritation or distress, perhaps even pain. The need to eliminate bodily wastes is also, obviously, an irritation and tension-producing situation that is followed by relief of this tension.

Psychoanalytic and biological theories state that the newborn enters this world with two basic drives. One is aggression, which provides a stimulus to obtain gratification. It is the drive that permits the baby to attempt to throw off intermittent states of overstimulation. The baby does this with the voluntary muscles. This kicking, clutching, and crying have the same components as what we later call tantrums; when the child is perhaps two years old, we begin to characterize this discharge of the irritation that the toddler finds overwhelming as "throwing a tantrum." Most of us react to this not as a signal of extreme distress as we did with the newborn but instead as the emotional blackmail of a "spoiled brat."

Similarly we almost always view such immature behavior in adults as obnoxious and perhaps dangerous. We rarely stop to consider where this pattern may have come from or what it actually means. Many cancer patients throw tantrums, but they do not seem to serve as a curative catharsis. However, this does indicate that these people are in a state of hyperirritation and are overwhelmed.

Aggression is usually viewed by people in general as a negative emotion. Most of us equate it with anger or hostility, but it does not have to be solely in the service of negative goals. For the newborn it may be used to make the baby's needs known—hardly a negative goal. Simply stated, aggression is a vital, necessary aspect of life, which must be integrated with other life-sustaining drives to help preserve a person.

The other drive that is viewed as innate is libido. In the Freudian sense, it is the force that motivates us to seek pleasure. Another way to view libido in the newborn is as the force that seeks tranquility. The baby is growing at an unbelievable rate. This growth, like healing, is believed by some to be painful and aggressive. A mending bone or a healing ulcer may cause pain, and both have cells that are reproducing rapidly to aid healing. Rapid mitotic growth (growth by cell division) in the newborn may also result in discomfort. The baby may be viewed as going through a healinglike process in all areas of her body. This physical and perhaps emotional pain must be dissipated or severe consequences can result. At times, nothing seems to work to dissipate it; but most of the time, the baby can gain relief through contact with others. Most frequently, this person is the mother. Libido in the newborn is simply the drive that seeks an escape from stimulation. The escape route is through the mother.

Margaret Mahler, an expert on early child development, calls this stage of life the "autistic stage." It usually lasts for the first two or three months of life and is the essence of self-containment. Mahler recognizes that growth is aggressive at this point in life and possibly even painful. And in the autistic stage, the baby has no ability to moderate the basic drives.

Thus, the baby may also be considered to be devoid of psychological defenses. It is the development of these defenses that marks the beginning of modulation of the drives. The newborn is the human being at the most sensitive, vulnerable, and impressionable stage of life.

We all have a tendency to ascribe far too mature feelings to this newcomer. We assume that the baby is angry when she is in fact letting us know that she is in a state of hyperirritation. We misunderstand the successful discharge of irritation as love. Because of our emotional needs, we attribute to the baby a far greater range of feelings than the baby is capable of. This also permits greater emotional attachment to the baby.

In reality, the baby cannot distinguish herself from her mother (or other caring individuals). Without something outside herself to attach irritation or pleasure to, the baby is not capable of rage or love. The baby is simply able to experience irritation or the lack of it.

In the course of the autistic stage the baby is conditioned into more advanced feelings. The parent (or surrogate) provides the conditioning to educate the child. Any kind of irritation in the autistic stage will bring forth outbursts of distress, including crying, flailing of arms and legs, and arching of the back. This unspecific reaction of the newborn to all irritation provides no clue as to the cause of the outburst and requires parental response based upon logic and knowledge of the baby's very limited physical and emotional needs.

A new parent's initial responses are likely to be based on trial and error, but the chances of successfully reducing irritation are very good because of the limited needs of the baby. After several weeks the parent will be able to respond to the baby's signals in a more direct, nonrandom manner. Once the mother can begin to tell what cry or movement relates to each need, then the baby is being conditioned to repeat the behavioral signals. If the baby does, gratification arrives much sooner. If the baby's mother does not become tuned in at this very early point in development, the baby will learn very little about giving off signals to be gratified or how to relate to the outside world.

This conditioning is on a physical sensate level only. It does not require thought or the ability to relate cause and effect; all it requires is an ability to feel, react, and be rewarded. This conditioning may involve thinking, but thought is not necessary for physical learning to take place. Single-cell organisms also have clearcut behaviors. Very primitive simple beings can apparently learn, that is, be conditioned. Even plants have responses (called tropisms) to stimuli, which indicate an ability to adapt.

The autistic stage of life is usually viewed as devoid of any great potential for learning, but recent observations have indicated that the newborn is more sensorially aware than previously assumed. However, the ability to take in from the environment is secondary to the lack of moderation of the drives. There is no learning within the sensory system that will help moderate the levels of hyperirritation until the conditioning takes place. The baby's intense ability to feel is indicative of the lack of such moderating psychological defenses.

It is this very rawness and immediate accessibility to aggression and libido that make the autistic-stage baby susceptible to unconscious learning mainly with the involuntary nervous system. This learning precedes consciousness, as we understand it, for the more mature individual. Autism appears to be a stage beyond cognitive or even emotional reach.

What can be conditioned in the first several weeks of life that will reduce tension resulting from irritation? If all goes well, it can be a wonderful lifelong degree of being comfortable with intimacy and in relating to others. If, right from the beginning, the baby has been taught how to be comfortable with unconditional loving, as an adult he will be accepting of such displays of caring directed at him.

If things do not go well, the learned response will be a dynamic for cancer. As an adult, this individual will reflect a basic trait that I have observed across the board in cancer patients. He will have developed all sorts of emotional defenses to prevent himself from being unconditionally loved and accepted. He will be uncomfortable, embarrassed, and sometimes even appear provoked if love is directed at him.

The newborn baby cannot condition himself. Whether or not the conditioning is excellent or horrendous, the care giver, usually the mother, is in a sense an involuntary participant. She can offer the baby only what her unconsciousness will permit. She can offer only what she has experienced and has been taught. She can offer only what her life circumstances will allow. Motherhood can be a joy. It is also a difficult job, which in our present society is far too frequently put down. Mothers are the individuals best suited for the early stage of rearing babies. The mothers cannot be perfect, but they cannot be substituted for either—not even by fathers.

Let me explain this highly controversial statement.

A great deal has been written about the emotional impact of pregnancy. For many women this is one of the most delightful times in their existence. However, one cannot deny that fear and discomfort are also significant aspects of carrying a child. Coupled with a lack of control over what is happening to one's body, they facilitate a vitally important regression.

Whether it is a first or a fifth pregnancy, it is very difficult for any woman to be really nonchalant about the situation. Having had several previous children may reduce fear to some degree, but each pregnancy represents a new unknown.

The first trimester of pregnancy is a shock to many emotional and physical systems. This serves as the initiator of the maternal regression. A feeling of being dissociated or "spaced out" is not infrequent. A hypersensitivity to irritation is also beginning. Certain smells and tastes may be repulsive; noise or glare may be more irritating than usual; touch may be experienced as abrasive at times.

By the second trimester, any ability to deny the pregnancy is taken away as it starts to show. The thought of not being able to say, "Okay guys, I've had enough. I think I'll just go home now," becomes a stark reality. The pregnancy is on a one-way street at this point. A very primitive feeling of vulnerability usually begins in the latter part of the second trimester as the abdomen enlarges and the future mother senses that her ability to fight or flee is greatly reduced.

Strange urges for food may be a result of this phenomenon. They are a test of the husband's willingness to be unconditionally giving and loving. A caring husband should never dismiss such requests as absurd. At this point, the 10:00 P.M. or 3:00 A.M. feeding of the baby is first taking place through the emotional and physical apparatus of the mother. She is unconsciously experimenting with the future. As her fears and loss of control over her body continue, she will regress more and more. And she will need frequent reassurance from her surrogate mother—her husband. Women are usually aware that they are testing at this point. As one woman reported:

> I asked Jim to go out and get me some ice cream last night. At 11:30 P.M. we were getting into bed when I felt like I had to have some vanilla fudge or I'd die. Jim had just gotten under the covers and turned out his light. I love him so much! He got right out of bed and got dressed to go get it. When he went out to the garage and turned on the car, I ran out and stopped him. I felt really crazy. I told him not to go, that the stores would all be closed. He said he knows an all-night deli that has ice cream. I told him I had changed my mind and didn't really want any. He sort of

shrugged, came over to me, hugged me, and said that I was a nut case but he loves me anyway. I felt so warm and cared for. I kissed him, and we went upstairs and made love.

By the third trimester, emotional changes are occurring at a rapid rate. Mood swings are more pronounced. Weepiness for no apparent reason can occur; an increase in hypersensitivity to all sorts of irritation may take place. The expectant mother is already experiencing many of the significant emotions that the newborn will experience. As pregnancy reaches its climax, the unborn baby and mother are remarkably similar in emotional orientation. At times the mother may feel she is losing control of her emotionality. The adult part of her psyche may condemn the emergence of infantile feelings; however, all of these feelings are both natural and necessary.

The more comfortable the woman is with her emotional state prior to pregnancy, the more supportive her marital relationship, the more likely it is that she will be able to be in touch with all her feelings during pregnancy. The more she can be in touch with all her feelings and express them, the more adequately she will regress to the baby's emotional level.

If the mother-to-be has a weak grasp of her feelings and reality prior to pregnancy, she will most likely resist regressing. She will fear permanently losing control of her emotions. At birth she and the baby will be at two very different emotional points.

After delivery our adult baby is both tired from physical exertion and emotional overstimulation. She may be euphoric and agitated simultaneously. She requires rest and soothing to regroup her forces. The highly volatile and extreme feelings of pregnancy will continue, and she will remain highly sensitive to irritation, both chemical and emotional.

In the next three months of the mother's and baby's life the emotional state of the mother may have enormous consequences for her child's future. How can these first three months be so important? Why are they more important in many regards than any stages in life? Why is the mother-baby interaction so vital for all later development? The answers to all of these questions can be provided through the concept of mother-baby fusion. It is this fusion, or lack of it, that makes the critical difference.

3

Fusion

THE PREVIOUS CHAPTER offered an explanation of how the mother and baby arrive at the same emotional point at the time of birth. She gets there through regression, and the baby gets there through intrauterine development. The mother's regression will permit a fusion or bonding between the baby and herself.

According to psychoanalytic theory, while pregnant the mother-to-be and her baby are viewed by her as being "one in the same." The baby is in the mother. The mother at the same time is emotionally in the baby. At birth, either the fusion of pregnancy continues and/or intensifies, or it abates. If the fusion is permitted and encouraged to continue and if it is sufficiently powerful, the mother will continue to function in and out of an autistic emotional state, the *primary maternal regression.* She will be experiencing infantile feelings and sensitivity at times, but she will also have the ability to use more mature defenses and function as a normal adult.

The truly beneficial aspects of the primary maternal regression center upon the mother's ability to feel like a baby. She will be one-half of the hypersensitive unity of mother and newborn. She may have extremes of feelings, which medical science explains in terms of hormone adjustments after delivery. Psychologically these extremes can be explained in terms of the normal infantile extremes of the autistic or first extrauterine stage of life. Some of the mysteries of the baby have ended. She can see, hear, touch, smell, and taste the baby, who now begins the lifelong process, which we call learning, of interpreting all these sensory clues.

If the mother cannot regress to the purity of feeling that pregnancy normally induces, she may be overwhelmed by the birth of her baby. She may feel disconnected from the strange creature with whom she has so little in common. If her regression stopped just short of autism, she will be at a point in emotional development called the anaclitic depression. This is an infantile depression that has nothing to do with more mature depression.* She is stuck at a point of regression in which she cannot tolerate the impingements of others. She wants to be alone and yet suffers extreme emotional pain if left alone. Postpartum depression can be in part or largely a resistance to fusion with the child.

In the treatment of precancerous and cancer patients, this concept of the infantile or anaclitic depression is vitally important. In chapter 12 I will have a great deal to say about it and about reversing it as a means of aiding in cancer treatment.

In most cases, the fusion will take place in pregnancy and continue for some time after birth. In terms of the beginning of cancer, fusion is most relevant during the first few months of life. The baby is the human being at his most vulnerable and impressionable state. Chemical and physical irritants from the inside and outside are helping to stimulate enormously rapid growth through cell division (mitosis). This process may at times be aggravating or even painful. When we consider that healing is

---

*Unlike more advanced depressions involving guilt and the need for punishment, the anaclitic depression merely indicates a need for distance and emotional self-containment. This will be explained entirely in chapter 12.

usually based upon mitotic growth and is usually painful, just imagine if every organ system in your body was experiencing the sensation of healing.

What prevents the newborn from exploding from such internal overstimulation? First, the wiring of the newborn's system has not yet been properly insulated throughout the body. This prevents her experiencing the intense discomfort that such focusing would cause. Second is the psychological concept of *emotional entropy*.

Picture a bowl of piping hot soup. If you place a spoon in it and get up from the table for a few moments, when you return and pick up the spoon that was left in the soup, the metal handle burns your hand. The heat energy from the soup has sought a balancing of energy forces between itself, the air, the table, the bowl, and the spoon. The ceramic bowl, air, and table are not as good conductors of heat as a metal spoon.

The system of hot soup and spoon is an entropic one. Heat (i.e., energy) seeks a balance. It goes from the area of greatest intensity to an area of less intensity until both are balanced out at a reduced level of intensity. An evenness or homeostasis results. This is a natural phenomenon of physical science. It is also a natural process in the psychological management of irritation for the infant.

If we change the hot soup to the baby and the metal spoon to the mother, the dissipation of autistic-stage irritation can easily be seen as occurring through the psychological fusion of the mother and baby. The soup heats up sufficiently, and the baby is obviously irritated. The source of irritation does not matter. The mother, because of her emotional investment in loving her baby, can be accurately considered an oversized room-temperature spoon. When the upset occurs in the baby, she is there to absorb it. The hot soup fits into the huge spoon, and the heat can be rapidly and efficiently absorbed and equalized throughout the system. Psychically, the mother and baby are one system at this point. This increases the efficiency of this emotional entropic reaction.

A fusion must be present to help facilitate the entropic reaction, but after frequent and intense irritations from the baby, the mother may herself be less patient. The spoon is absorbing too much heat.

This is most likely to happen if the mother starts off irritated, with her emotional needs not being met by significant others (her husband or her parents, for example). The better she is cared for, the better she will be able to care for the baby. The cooler the spoon, the more it can absorb. The mother's irritations should be absorbed and dissipated by caring and concerned loved ones. If these people want to help and love the new baby to the greatest degree possible, they will first meet the new mother's emotional needs. She is the priority.

What happens if there are aberrations of this phenomenon of emotional entropy? If, the baby is consistently left to cry out his irritation on his own, the entropic soup-spoon system becomes totally self-contained. The baby will begin to learn all sorts of mechanisms to keep things in, right from the beginning of life. The state of *oneness* can actually kill.

The physiology of the newborn is highly vulnerable. As cells rapidly reproduce, they are vulnerable to a process of genetic shifting that may have severe consequences immediately if the self-containment is extreme. More likely the biology will be thrown slightly out of whack in terms of future susceptibility to irritation.

The death of babies from marasmus is not the same as Sudden Infant Death (SID) syndrome. SID apparently results from a neurological defect that causes the baby to stop breathing. With marasmus the baby shows lethargy, passivity, and refusal to fuse with others prior to dying from "no apparent physical causes." Marasmus is the most extreme reaction to lack of emotional entropy between mother and child.

According to studies, we know that the risk of marasmus increases if the mother is less than twenty years old, is unmarried, poor, and has had no prenatal care. The risk is higher among the lower social and economic levels of our society. Those least at risk are Asian Americans, while poor Blacks are at the other extreme. Significantly, twins and triplets run a greater risk than single births. Boys are more frequently victims than girls. What all this adds up to is that life circumstances that prevent a primary maternal regression and subsequent fusion with the newborn appear to relate directly to marasmus.

The next step down from marasmus in severity is a conditioning for childhood autism or schizophrenia. Children are diagnosed as autistic, while adults with similar symptoms are usually referred to as schizophrenic. To avoid confusion, while still using the accepted terminology, I will from this point onward refer to childhood autism of a pathological degree as childhood schizophrenia. It cannot be diagnosed in an autistic-stage child. It refers to the youngster who never leaves this stage.

The child behaves as if there is no outside world. He is incapable of responding to other people. He is incapable of protecting himself from dangers in his environment and usually does not even develop an adequate means of communication with anyone else. He has avoided developing a concept of the other as a means of defending himself against a fear of being overwhelmed by the significant other.

The schizophrenic child is one who seems, in effect, to have turned off his mental apparatus in order to tolerate nurturing by an unconsciously hostile, perhaps even murderous, mother. She does not act maliciously or abusively. She has no conscious intent of doing the baby harm. As a matter of fact, she may be obsessive about doing all the right things. *She is not a voluntary contributor to the problem. In a sense she is as much a victim as the infant. Blaming her for her unconscious rage toward her baby would be like blaming people for what they dream.* Her need to do everything

43

right, to be the perfect mother, is a means of denying this unconscious rage.

Mothers of schizophrenic children do all the right things. Consciously they feel all the right things. It is only the tip of the iceberg, however, that we see; the one-eighth of the mass that is above the surface represents the conscious feelings of the new mother. It is the seven-eighths below the surface that the baby can sense far more readily than adults. Babies, animals, and schizophrenics can tune into unconscious feelings like long-range radar detectors. No one can hide unconscious feelings from a baby. We have all seen babies scream whenever certain people come near.

The newborn has a limited means of escape from a mother with unconscious hostile feelings. Physically he certainly cannot escape. But mentally he can resist and, thus, sacrifice learning to relate emotionally to this significant figure.

Schizophrenia, in my opinion, results from dissipating irritation to avoid marasmus. The mental apparatus is sacrificed to prevent death caused by overwhelming emotional irritation.

Do not forget that emotional irritation results in chemical change in all stages of human life. Keep in mind also that a state of hyperirritation can result in a possible overwhelming number of genetic shifts in the rapidly dividing cells.

Psychoanalysts are still being taught that if a person's mind is insane then his cells cannot be insane, that is, cancerous. The theory is that the mind is attacked rather than the body. The internalized rage, as the analysts would see this primitive response to irritation, is stored in the mind instead of the body. This is a nice, neat formula for entropic shifting within a self-contained individual. Schizophrenics are certainly self-contained. Whether they are children or adults, the fixation at the autistic stage is very easily discernible.

According to this theory, schizophrenics should not develop cancer. But while working at a state hospital in New York, I saw many actively schizophrenic patients who had cancer, and there was no apparent difference between the cancers of normal people and schizophrenics.

Schizophrenia is not an alternative to cancer. It is only an alternative to marasmus.

As the child attempts to turn off the unconscious hostile feelings of his mother, he is learning to turn off the entire world for the mother is the newborn's entire world. When the baby should be developing a connection, the person he is to connect to is far too frightening. Thus, the baby stays within himself. While this basic dynamic for schizophrenia is designed to limit the baby's sensitivity to his environment to prevent overwhelming degrees of irritation, this defense does not achieve its intended purpose. If the baby really could turn off all his awareness of his mother, he would be living his early life in a totally fusionless state, which would result in marasmus. Instead the future schizophrenic can still dissipate some irritation to the outside, to mother. Thus he can learn factual things and even survive in a hostile world as an adult. But to do so necessitates that he allow sufficient irritation inward to establish chemical changes and thus genetic shifting. The predisposing factors for future cancer are thus established.

Schizophrenia is an inefficient adjustment. If, as most theories postulate, the purpose of schizophrenia is to contain rage and screen out the fear object, or mother, it fails miserably at its task while permitting the dynamics for all sorts of psychosomatic disorders.

Schizophrenic adults and children are aware of a great many of the irritations and stimulations that impinge upon them. They are aware of chemical irritation to a far greater extent than most of us. Their mental apparatus hallucinates smells, tastes, touches, and, more commonly, sights and sounds so that they may continue the sensations of early infancy in an unconscious attempt to undo them. We all hold onto what is familiar rather than do what is best for us. We may be doing this as a means of expressing our desire for someone to fuse to who can repeat the original mistakes.

Like cancer, schizophrenia does run in families. But like cancer, it can be viewed as a learned characteristic passed on from one generation to the next. The fact that schizophrenics can be treated successfully with modern psychoanalysis tends to devalue the theory that it is hereditary.

Cancer, like schizophrenia, is a defense against marasmus. In schizophrenia, the attempt to dissipate hyperirritation is through the mind. In cancer, the hyperirritation that does not get adequately dissipated during early infancy is stored in the body cells, perhaps through the process of genetic translocation or shifting of the position of the genes along the chromosome (this will be explained in chapter 4). At the same time a conditioning takes place in the mind and body to maximize irritation, to be self-contained, and to view life as a basically irritating experience.

Cancer is seemingly the baby's least severe reaction to an overwhelming degree of irritation. The result is not immediate. The genetic shifting and psychological conditioning that predisposes the individual to cancer later on in life is a slow process. Let us examine how it happens.

We start off with mother and baby as a twosome once again. In this case, the mother has successfully regressed to the baby's emotional level, and the emotional entropy (soup-spoon) is operating well. When the baby feels irritated, the mother soothes him, and the irritation goes from his involuntary nervous system to her. The baby's cells continue dividing rapidly in a normal, healthy way.

But if the mother periodically adds powerfully to the baby's irritation or does nothing to siphon it off, the dynamics for cancer, both biologically and psychologically, will be established. Rather than be overwhelmed and have cells die from irritation, or succumb to marasmus, the irritation is channeled into the baby's very core to be stored as a translocated gene ready to be activated in the face of additional subsequent irritation. Cancer is thus stored as a land mine implanted in the individual. The shift in genes is the bomb with its detonator set to go off. All that is necessary is for sufficient irritation in the future to trigger the explosion.

The question arises as to why the baby does not immediately develop cancer. The answer is that in the autistic stage of life, the baby's cells would first have to translocate, then become malignant, and then be diagnosed. All of this may take months or years to happen. According to Dr. Rita Harper, Chief of Neonatology at North Shore University Hospital in New York, almost no babies are born with cancer. This and Greene's identical twin study should help reduce fear that cancer is hereditary.

The development of cancer is at least a two-step proposition. First activator genes are stimulated next to the gene that will later shift. This probably occurs in infancy. The activator gene stores the cells' ability to respond to irritation by reproducing through cell division. This may be the normal biological dissipation of irritation in infancy.

If after the irritation, the new mother soothes and comforts the baby, the cells that reproduce will now be normal, and the land mine will be surrounded by healthy tissue.

If a fluctuation of feeling is predominately the style of a mother's interaction with her newborn, more and more land mines will be laid down. Unfortunately this is how many children are raised. But if love and caring predominate and if the episodes of unsoothed hyperirritation are few and short-lived, the baby will have a far better chance of never developing cancer because of fewer initial stage translocations occurring.

The mother's communication of irritation does not have to be conscious or direct. Her unconscious irritation is far more devastating. Babies are magnets for unconscious feelings. Any mother who can admit to herself that she feels hostility toward her new baby at times is less likely to set up the dynamics of cancer. It is when she does not want to know, probably because she does not trust her impulses, that the baby is at the greatest risk. This is when the land mines are laid down and a psychological conditioning is established to maximize irritation throughout life. Remember that we do not do what is best for us, we do what is familiar. If from the beginning of life the baby has been conditioned to add irritation to existing irritation, he will maintain this hypersensitivity to all irritants throughout life. Whether these carcinogens are emotional, directly chemical, or physical is unimportant. Any one of them can activate the land mine. If no genetic translocation occurred in the earliest stages of life, then the responses to irritation will be other psychosomatic disorders. If genetic shifts could occur in utero, then babies would be born with cancer.

To recapitulate:

1. The most severe disorder caused by lack of or incomplete fusion is marasmus. This occurs because of the emotional-chemical irritations of infancy remaining within an almost totally self-contained system within the baby's body.

2. The intermediate alternative to infantile death from irritation is schizophrenia. In this case, the mental apparatus gets sacrificed in an attempt to ward off irritation from the outside. It does not work, and thus schizophrenics can develop cancer.

3. The least severe consequence of intermittent hyperirritation is the establishment of biological and psychological dynamics for future cancer. This is a delaying tactic that prevents infantile death from hyperirritation. It is so extremely internalized that it goes unnoticed in small children. More developed communication ability is necessary for the precancerous state to be discernible.

The following hypothetical case histories, based upon people I have known and studies pertaining to the relevant facts, will help to clarify these stages of development.

Fusion

Brian

Emily is twenty-two years old and single. She lives in a large city in the East. She has been employed as a factory worker, a domestic, and an office cleaning woman. She does not hold jobs very long. At the time of the birth of her fourth child, this petite, attractive woman was unemployed and had no man in her life. Emily's family lives in the South; she has had no contact with them since she ran away at the age of sixteen with a local boy who became the father of her firstborn, a son named Charles. Each of her children was fathered by a different man. Maintaining relationships is not one of Emily's fortes; she does not even consider it an issue in her life.

Almost every year that she has been away from her parents, she has become pregnant. Prior to the birth of her fourth baby, Brian, she had two daughters. She also miscarried just prior to Brian's conception.

Emily drinks wine and beer to excess. She rationalizes that getting drunk this way is all right because she is not drinking hard liquor. No one ever told her not to drink during pregnancy; no one ever told her anything during pregnancy. She has never had prenatal care.

Six-year-old Charles already clearly manifests serious problems. He shows almost no emotion, regardless of the circumstances. He does what he is told when he is told. The two girls, Mary and Elizabeth, seem relatively emotionally stable and bright. Emily candidly admits that girl babies were always easier for her to care for. She talks of dressing them in the cutest outfits she can afford.

As newborns, the boys cried all the time. Charles stopped crying when he was about eight months old. He has almost never cried since. Brian stopped crying almost totally when he was about four months old. He stopped crying completely when he died at the age of five months three weeks.

After Brian's birth, Emily was unable to care for him properly.

She was depressed and agitated. When he cried, she could not stand it. She was afraid to pick him up because she was worried about dropping him. Emily knew that her inability to care for Brian meant that something was very wrong, so she followed the advice of a very nice concerned nurse and attended a free post-natal care course given in a city hospital. The nurse practitioner who taught the course immediately diagnosed her as being in a postpartum depression. She recommended that Emily see one of the psychiatric social workers. At this suggestion, Emily flew into a rage, protesting that she was not crazy and did not need a "Goddamned shrink." She stormed out of the classroom and never returned. She taught Charles how to care for his baby brother, and she devoted herself to her girls.

Once when Brian was two weeks old and crying, Emily could not stand his behavior; she placed him and his carriage in the bathroom and closed the door. Brian cried for an hour and a half before he fell asleep. From that time on, the baby's crying resulted in solitary confinement.

By the age of four months, strangers felt uncomfortable with him. His facial expression was bland and sad. If anyone approached him, he looked away. If he was picked up, he cried, then screamed, then went rigid in the hands that held him. He was not a pleasant child to be near. No one wanted to hold him.

At five months of age he began to lose weight. Then one night while he was sleeping in the bathroom, while his mother was out with friends and while little Charles was asleep, Brian died. Emily came home at four in the morning. She was not going to even risk waking him by opening the bathroom door. When she decided on second thought to look, she saw what she thought was a sleeping baby. Charles found his half brother at 7:00 A.M. He woke his mother with tears in his eyes.

The cause of death was listed as marasmus. There was an autopsy, and the pathologists could find no physical cause of death. Brian became another statistic in the research annals of marasmus.

Brian died from a total lack of love.

Lorraine

Janet and Michael have a shaky marriage. Their only reason for marrying was Janet's pregnancy. Michael is an attorney who spends most of his off-hours on the golf course. His firm specializes in corporate law, and it is not uncommon for Michael to work until midnight. Janet was aware of this when she married him, but she also believed that she could at least break him of his fanatic obsession with golf.

Janet was working as a paralegal in Michael's firm when they began dating. She had been an elementary school teacher for one year when she decided that she honestly could not tolerate all of those children at once. She had resorted to strict discipline, and, of course, a revolution ensued.

In general, people describe Janet as a nice "girl" who is a bit too high-strung. In reality, Janet, a perfectionist, becomes very upset when she thinks things are not right in her world. A slightly overcooked dinner is a disaster. She is obsessed by the fact that she gained quite a lot of weight after her pregnancy, but she fails miserably at dieting.

Before the baby was born, she decided that Michael's dog had to go because it was dirty. Her cat was moved from inside to outside. Any room in the house could be used as an emergency operating room.

Janet insists on doing things on time. She is the kind of person who becomes livid if someone else is late. She is always at least five minutes early. She is intolerant about most things. Heaven help the person who lights up a cigarette near her in a restaurant.

Janet has few friends, and her in-laws dislike her. She makes people feel uncomfortable. She is aware of this, although no one has talked to her about it. Her anger is just below the surface, just below the awareness of herself and others. Something is just not right about her.

Janet's parents are both dead. Her mother died of lymphoma when Janet was seventeen. The year before her wedding, her father died, in a private psychiatric hospital, of a heart attack. He had been in and out of psychiatric facilities most of Janet's life. He was totally withdrawn during her formative years.

Before the baby was born, Janet read everything she could find about child care. She knew all of the psychological theories about intrauterine development, birth, and early childhood. She decided that her child should be brought into the world correctly. She and Michael took Lamaze training. But after four hours of labor, she could not persevere and accepted demerol and scopolamine. The baby, Lorraine, was healthy and weighed in at nine pounds two ounces.

Breastfeeding was advocated in the Lamaze classes, but Janet complained of discomfort and inconvenience. The baby's loose bowel movements, normal in early breastfeeding, nauseated her every time she had to change Lorraine.

Janet felt that she had failed a significant test of womanhood, "natural childbirth," when Lorraine was born. Unconsciously she condemned Lorraine for being so large and thus setting her up for failure. When she was unsuccessful at breastfeeding, she consciously blamed herself. But under the surface, she believed that Lorraine was insatiable and would suck her very life away. She tried demand feeding, and again failure ensued because she was not tuned in to the baby's needs. Success came, she thought, when she resorted to scheduled feeding. Her pediatrician told her to adhere rigidly to the schedule and let the baby cry. Rigid adherence to schedules was something Janet was used to and enjoyed. At times she let Lorraine cry herself to sleep hungry.

When she cared for the baby physically, she attempted to hide her hostile feelings beneath a facade of sweetness and gentility; when Lorraine cried, Janet felt slapped in the face.

When Janet felt too upset, she would put the baby down. On occasion she would scream at her newborn to shut up, but that was rare. Most of the time, she just felt uncomfortable with the baby.

It never occurred to her that she was entitled to some time off away from the baby, that she needed a break. To her, this would have been another admission of failure. Michael was also no help and made it clear that the stress of his job was overwhelming him. Whenever she spoke of any feelings, he retreated. Janet was alone raising her baby, a horrendous situation for anyone.

She first noticed Lorraine's lack of interest in outside objects when she was about eight months of age. Lorraine was already an extremist in reaction to stimulation. She either screamed or was indifferent. There was no middle ground.

By three years of age, Lorraine had still not learned to speak. She sat for long periods rocking back and forth, apparently oblivious to whatever went on around her. If anyone touched her, she flinched. If she was picked up, she screamed and pushed away. She would shake her hands as if trying to get something off that was stuck to them. Lorraine was diagnosed by several different psychiatrists and psychologists as being a childhood schizophrenic, an autistic child. She had never emotionally left the first stage of life. Her mother's unconsciously hostile feelings toward her resulted in Lorraine's sacrificing her mental apparatus in order to become insensitive to this additional irritation. She was using a psychobiological defense, which attempts to accomplish the same thing that Thorazine will do, against her mother's unconsciously hostile feelings. She was cutting down on the irritation from the outside so that it could not add to the irritation from the inside. Lorraine learned to turn off the outside world.

By the age of five, Lorraine and her parents were receiving

professional help, but Janet remained convinced that nothing would work. For her, that may be tragically true. For Lorraine, a corrective reexperiencing of the autistic stage seems to be permitting her emotions to mature. Her therapists spend hours forcing her to pay attention to them. She was at first terrified of their coercion. But when she began to realize somehow that they would not add to her irritation but soothe it instead, she began to allow them in. Her therapists also understand that her apparent fits of rage are really an expression of hyperirritation from an infantile stage. There is good cause for optimism for this little girl.

Alice

Susan was thirty-five when she conceived for the third time. She wanted a boy. Her husband said he did not care. Half-jokingly she told him he would have to make up for this one by agreeing to another pregnancy if this baby were a girl.

Susan and John had been married for nine years at this time. Their eldest child was a boy of seven named Robert. The second child was a three-year-old named Mary Ann.

Susan did a lot of caring for others during this pregnancy. Robert had frequent bouts with ear infections, which responded to antibiotics but flared up again after brief respites. Her husband seemed somewhat detached, although he did occasionally go out for midnight ice cream cones. He complained about her lack of interest in sex, which predated the pregnancy and was exacerbated by it. John argued that he could not be as giving as he would like unless Susan showed some consideration for his needs, but he complimented her on how differently she was behaving in all other regards during this pregnancy. At times, when she seemed to be off in her own world, he retreated to his hobby of making furniture.

Her labor and delivery went well. She went to the hospital four hours prior to delivering Alice. Intense labor lasted for less than an hour, and she required no drugs. Susan decided not to breast-feed because of the inconvenience it caused. She did part-time work in her husband's store and wanted to return as soon as possible.

Alice was an adorable baby, and even though Susan regretted that she was not a boy, she related well to her. But she did have a mild feeling of depression that lasted for two weeks after the birth.

With this baby, they decided to have no live-in help. John's mother had come to assist them after the births of the first two children, but this time Susan assured John that she could handle everything herself. For the most part, she could, even though Robert's ear infections continued, Mary Ann behaved just like any other four-year-old, and John remained unaffectionate, although he assisted with looking after the children.

The pediatrician remarked on Alice's beauty and apparent good health, but he did express concern for Susan's depleted look. He recommended a blood workup and urine analysis. He counseled her to take proper care of herself.

During Alice's fifth week of life, she, for no apparent reason, started waking up more often during the night. Susan suspected that something was wrong, but the doctor gave Alice a clean bill of health and brushed off the sudden change in her sleep cycle as one of the things modern medicine did not have an explanation for. Susan thought irritably to herself that they probably did not even think about the issue. She felt that science had better things to investigate than why babies wake up for no apparent reason.

On Alice's first wakeful night, Susan had been sympathetic and concerned. She sat and walked holding her baby, noticing how small and fragile looking this tiny human was. She studied her little fingers, amazed at their perfection. The tiny nails fascinated her. As Alice settled down, her hands and feet stopped the random movements of an irritated baby. Their eyes met just prior to the baby falling asleep in Susan's arms. A glow permeated every inch of Susan. She was in love with her baby. She sat staring at her for fifteen minutes, watching her facial expressions change. There was something almost mystical about this fusion, and Susan did not want to break the spell. When she finally put Alice back in her crib, the baby twitched a little bit as her mother's hand left her back. Susan immediately placed her hand gently on the baby again. Alice slept peacefully for the rest of the night.

By the fourth night, the mysticism was gone; so was the fusion. When Alice woke up screaming, Susan shuddered. She rolled over in bed and tried to follow her own reasonable five-minute rule. If the baby did not stop crying in five minutes, she would get up. Susan was enraged at being awakened again. All she wanted to do was sleep like John, who was out to the world. It was his busy season, and she felt much too guilty to wake him.

After three minutes, she leaped out of bed, put her robe on, and stormed into the nursery. She grabbed Alice and changed her. She realized that she was very upset, but she would not blame this adorable baby for it. She held Alice while trying to control and deny her desire to kill her. Alice continued to be obviously irritated, but she soon stopped crying in the presence of such irritation from her mother. The containment was no longer just self-containment. *Alice* was absorbing *Susan*'s irritation entropically.

This irritation immediately translated to self-produced chemical irritants. The activator gene was switched to the *on* position to permit subsequent genetic shifts of a sort that have been directly related to many forms of cancer, for example, urinary bladder, breast, lung, lymphoma, bone, and numerous other cancers.

At the very same instant, Susan was teaching Alice to hold her feelings in when she was hyperirritated. She was teaching her to be resistant to the unconditional expressions of love that should be part of everyone's life. She was teaching her to resist fusion as a means of dissipating irritation throughout her life. Alice would

56

grow up to seek out people she could care for rather than allow herself any conscious desire, which would be too dangerous, to have childlike or infantile needs.

An hour later, Susan was lying awake in bed, still very upset and guilty about her reactions to Alice but calming herself down. Unable to sleep, she went to check on Alice. She picked her up gently. Again the mysticism of the fusion was obvious. Alice's cells were now dividing in a normal healthy way, surrounding the pretranslocation cells of the episode of hyperirritation. The land mine was buried and hidden. Fluctuations like this occurred throughout the early months of Alice's life.

Thirty-nine years later, Alice was married and had grown children. She worked for a textile company and was exposed to various chemicals used in the dyeing process. Her nineteen-year-old son was serving as a helicopter gunner in the U.S. Marines. When out drinking with a friend, her son was in an accident. The car was demolished. He was killed.

Alice was overcome with grief. Her husband turned to alcohol and other women. Ten months after her son's death and her husband's falling apart, she was diagnosed as having pancreatic cancer. Emotional and chemical carcinogens had triggered the translocation that was set up in infancy.

As her cancer progressed, Alice became more and more infantile. She eventually had to be fed, became incontinent, and could not walk. She was unable to think clearly or, eventually, even to speak. She cried pathetically. Her body and mind had returned to total autism. Two years after her diagnosis, Alice died at the chronological age of forty-one. Her emotional age was close to zero.

All three of these people are examples of the consequences of aberrations of the maternal-infant bond.

4

Biological Concepts
of the Causes of Cancer:
Genetics and Virology

Genetics

IT IS AS WRONG TO DENY relevant genetic laws as it is to blame them for disorders we do not understand. Cancer is genetic in origin. It is, however, not hereditary. A knowledge of the basics of genetic theory is all that is required to understand this seemingly contradictory statement.

Most of the ten trillion cells that make up the human body have a nucleus that contains genes, the basic carriers of hereditary traits. These genes are organized as strands called chromosomes. (Red blood cells are a notable exception in that they have no nuclei or genetic material.) Each gene is made up of the chemical DNA, deoxyribonucleic acid. We know about the structure of DNA molecules, chromosomal aberrations, and dominant and recessive genes and still cannot explain cancer based on this knowledge.

When cells reproduce in our bodies, one of two things happens. If they are reproducing to become egg or sperm through oogenesis or spermatogenesis, the end result will be cells (ova or sperm)

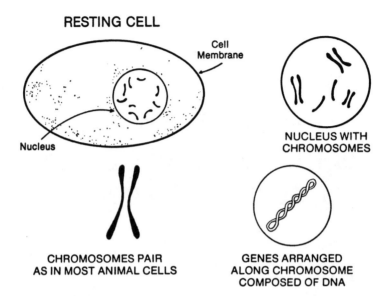

RESTING CELL

Cell
Membrane

Nucleus

NUCLEUS WITH
CHROMOSOMES

CHROMOSOMES PAIR
AS IN MOST ANIMAL CELLS

GENES ARRANGED
ALONG CHROMOSOME
COMPOSED OF DNA

with half the normal complement of chromosomes and genes. When fertilization takes place, the fertilized egg has the full complement. This mixing of half-complements makes us all genetically unique, with the exception of identical twins, who evolve from the same fertilized eggs.

Even siblings, while frequently similar in many observable physical (phenotypic) regards, are remarkably different in genetic endowment (genotypic).

The other type of cell reproduction is through simple cell division. Almost all cells not slated for reproduction of the organism reproduce genetic material and divide. This is called mitosis. A notable exception are neurons (nerve cells).

The cells synthesize or break down chemical compounds, which are necessary for metabolic processes. Some organ systems have cells that reproduce more rapidly than others. These include hair follicles and the lining of the digestive tract. The divided cells function exactly as their predecessors to serve a useful purpose.

Cancer cells do not. Cancer cells function only to replicate. They do not create or break down chemical compounds as do normal cells. They rob the body of nutrients and reproduce only cancer cells. (It takes only thirty cell divisions to produce a pea-sized cancer composed of up to a billion cells.)

Over three decades ago, Barbara McClintock presented a

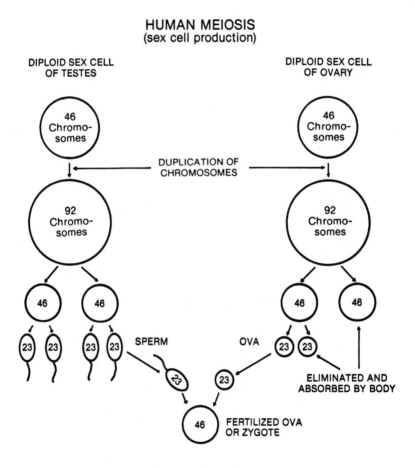

HUMAN MEIOSIS
(sex cell production)

seminar at the Cold Spring Harbor Laboratory on Long Island. Her topic was genetic translocation in corn.

She was largely ignored for years, but she continued her work independently. Relatively recently, others have studied genetic translocations in mammals. In March 1983, McClintock won Israel's Wolf Foundation Award. She also has won other significant scientific awards, including the Albert Lasker Basic Medical Research Award. Since 1946, thirty-three Lasker Award winners

MITOSIS — CELL DIVISION
(non-sex cell production)

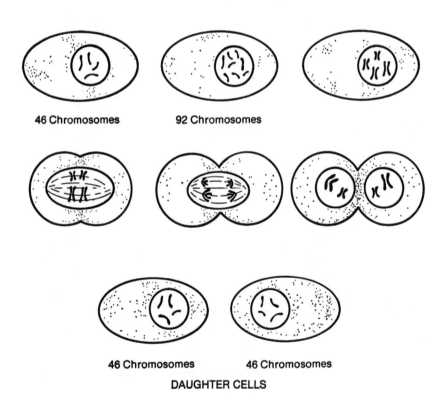

46 Chromosomes   92 Chromosomes

46 Chromosomes   46 Chromosomes
DAUGHTER CELLS

have subsequently received the Nobel Prize, as did McClintock in 1983.

Genetic translocation became the answer to a puzzling phenomenon McClintock observed in sweet corn (white or yellow). Corn, Zea maize in scientific terms, is the same species whether it is sweet corn or the colorful Indian corn of Thanksgiving. The difference in coloration in corn is caused by a few genes. The color changes seemed unimportant to many, but this phenomenon provided McClintock with a clue to something basic and fundamental to the science of genetics. She discovered that it was caused by a change in the chromosomal ordering of the genes. The string of genes that compose the chromosomes was not the rigidly ordered strand of beads the scientific community assumed it to be. Upon microscopic examination, she found that the genes had shifted from one position to another. The genes were "jumping."

The color, purple for instance, remained constant if the genes were left undisturbed. But after a "shock," genetic elements (genes) jumped or translocated to a position alongside the purple gene. The next generation of that kernel produced golden brown or bronze-colored kernels.

McClintock's work has already been used to explain how bacteria rapidly become immune to an antibiotic, how hereditary diseases occur, and how evolution itself may have taken place. It can also be used to explain cancer.

Keep in mind some of the more relevant facts of her discovery:

1. Genes can shift position along chromosomes.

2. A shock is necessary to activate the process (e.g., antibiotics are a shock to bacteria).

3. Too much of a shock could result in too much shifting for the cell to survive.

Genetic translocation can be viewed as a two-stage proposition. First, the irritation results in the activator gene becoming activated. Then the neighboring gene, or blob of DNA, jumps position. The activator stage may occur in infancy.*

The genetic shift may occur in response to later irritation. However, it is possible that the entire shift occurs in infancy and that further irritation later in life triggers this gene to cause rapid cell division. For simplicity's sake, I will refer to the infantile change and the adult precancerous biological posture as a genetic translocation.

In support of this application of translocation is the recent work of Weinberg,** Scolnick, and Lowry. They found such a switch in urinary bladder cancer. One nucleitide (gene) out of thousands was detected as being out of place in the malignant cells.

In the case of marasmus, repeated shocks to the nuclei and genetic material possibly result in overwhelming numbers of completed translocations, which have not been discernible to medical science in the search for a physical cause for such infant deaths.

In the less severe or shorter term states of hyperirritation, it is possible that only the activator stage gets triggered. Or, perhaps, far fewer translocations occur; this would throw off biological function so slightly as to be unnoticed.

At the beginning of life, most of the organ systems are undergoing rapid growth through cell division. At birth, the lungs, for

---

*The process that permits irritation to be transformed into stored energy is most probably the biochemical phenomenon of phosphorylation. All living organisms possess the chemical compound adenosine triphosphate (ATP). ATP is capable of storing large amounts of energy. If, under the influence of biochemical irritation, ATP gives off a phosphate group, this group can attach itself to the amino acids of a nucleotide. The receptive amino acids must have an available hydroxyl group (OH) for the bonding. The phosphate on this amino acid is then a potentially volatile source of sudden energy. This could account for the instability of nucleic material since a detonator has now been placed in the land mine.

**Weinberg, R., 1983.

64

GENETIC TRANSLOCATION

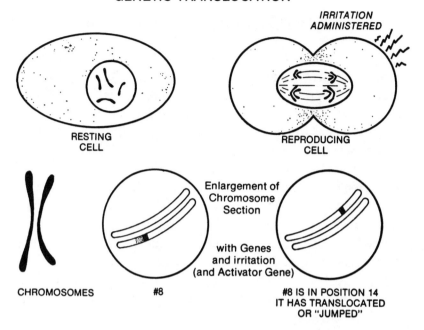

RESTING
CELL

IRRITATION
ADMINISTERED

REPRODUCING
CELL

CHROMOSOMES

#8

Enlargement of
Chromosome
Section

with Genes
and irritation
(and Activator Gene)

#8 IS IN POSITION 14
IT HAS TRANSLOCATED
OR "JUMPED"

example, have only 10 percent of the alveoli (air sacs) that the fully developed lungs will have. The gastrointestinal linings are still forming, as is the liver, endocrine systems, bones, etc. Everything is growing extremely rapidly through a process referred to as neoplasia.

Other types of growing processes and growth spurts can take place later in life. If an individual desires to enlarge his or her biceps or other muscles, growth can be accomplished through exercise. The exercise results in growth through the individual cells getting larger, not through an increased rate of cell reproduction. This type of growth is technically referred to as hypertrophy. It is not relevant to cancer. Neoplasia is.

You have probably heard that if the rate of growth in the first few months of life were to continue unabated, we would all end up the size of the Empire State Building. Just consider what might happen if such a rapid growth rate were to be somehow reactivated at a later time in life.

Cancer is a rapid and random reproduction of cells that function only to reproduce and steal nutrients from the body. Suppose that cancer is a reactivation of the rapid cell division of infancy, but, because the organ systems have already been formed, the cells have no place to go. Instead they form malignancies. When a tumor reaches maximum holding capacity for the cancer cells, spreading or metastasizing of the cancer follows.

If one looks at cancer cells through a microscope, one sees that they resemble the organ cells from which they originate. They are, however, misshapen and distorted in appearance.

If one fractures a bone or develops an ulcer, cells are activated toward rapid mitotic growth through the irritation of the injury and the influence of hormones. This is part of the normal healing process. But, in the case of cancer, healing is not the object. Growth becomes an end in itself.

Cancer is infantile growth and adult healing gone astray. Cancer is a reactivated infantile neoplasia with no place to go. This reactivation is caused by carcinogens, both chemical and emotional.

Virology

With a viral disease such as yellow fever, probably everyone bitten by a carrier mosquito gets the disease. In the case of another viral disease, the "common cold," infectivity is, believe it or not, rather low. In one study in England, only ten percent of the individuals exposed to other people suffering at the height of a cold contracted the infection. Measles, mumps, and chicken pox add to the list of apparently puzzling facts about viral effects. Once you get these illnesses, you are usually immune for the rest of your life.

Cancer is like none of these viral diseases. We all get bitten by the "carrier mosquitos" of cancer (namely, stress, chemical pol-lutants, X rays, etc.), but we do not all get cancer. No one on a hospital oncology (cancer) unit walks around attempting to guard against viral infection; doctors and nurses do not even wear masks or gowns. And if one is unfortunate enough to contract cancer, this certainly does not provide future immunity. Instead, the risks of recurrence are great.

When a bacterial infection is underway, the cells are sur-rounded by these "germs," which feed upon them. Bacteria are highly vulnerable to antibodies because they remain outside the cell. When a viral infection is taking place, however, the virus *enters* the cell and causes the genetic material in the cell to reproduce more of the same virus. Once inside the cell, antibodies have no effect upon the virus.

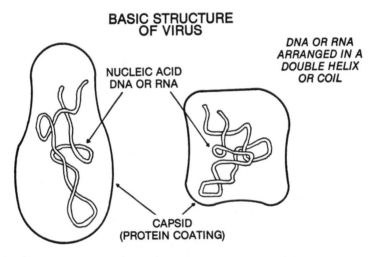

BASIC STRUCTURE
OF VIRUS

NUCLEIC ACID
DNA OR RNA

DNA OR RNA
ARRANGED IN A
DOUBLE HELIX
OR COIL

CAPSID
(PROTEIN COATING)

In discussing genetics, I mentioned DNA, which makes up the genes. DNA also makes up the core of the viruses. This genetic material found in viruses is also found in cancer cells, but most important, it is also found in normal cells. These substances can be inactivated in many cases by certain enzymes. But unfortunately, the DNA or RNA, which is synthesized by the DNA, in viruses is not readily accessible to enzymes because this material is encapsulated in a protective protein coating. This viral protein (antigen) induces the body to make specific antibodies, which will attack only viruses in that family. The coil of DNA or RNA (nucleic acids) is encased in the protein coating like a spring in a box waiting to pop out. The encapsulating protein coating of the container or boxlike formation is called a capsid. Interestingly, this protein coating is very similar to the chemical makeup of the cell membrane. But, by being *outside* the cell structure, the body now views it as a foreign protein or antigen; and therefore antibodies are produced, even though the membranes are similar.

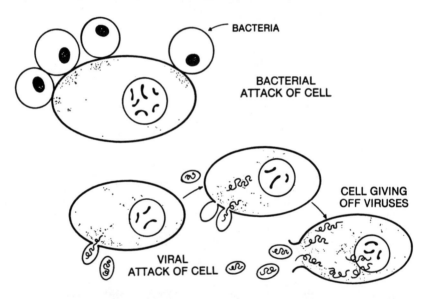

Viruses attach themselves to the cell membrane and, like a sperm on an egg cell, dissolve the membrane and inject the nucleic acids into the cells. The virus is like a hyperdermic needle; the material being injected is the nucleic acid, and the capsid is the syringe.

There are two major theories as to the evolution of viruses. The first is the Green-Laidlow hypothesis* that follows: All creatures who lead basically parasitic lives discard structures and functions that are unnecessary for survival. Fleas, which are related to flies, have lost their wings. Tapeworms have no alimentary (digestive) canal because they absorb nutrients through their exteriors. Viruses, according to Green and Laidlow, may have evolved from malaria parasites, protozoa, or bacteria.

Another hypothesis presented by C. H. Andrewes,** is that viruses are produced from the cell's own nucleic acid. Again, however, it is assumed that some irritant from the outside first enters the cell to stimulate the liberation of DNA or RNA. It then can be expelled, receiving a protective coating of protein from the cell membrane as it is on its way out. The virus is suddenly present without there having been any apparent cause of infection.

This no "apparent cause of infection" is most important. Suppose this second evolutionary process could take place: a cell that had suffered from a translocation (jumping gene) is somehow stimulated to expel the translocated nucleic acid of the gene fragment. As it leaves the cell membrane, it is coated with protein, and we have nucleic acid enclosed in a capsid, in other words a virus.

Virus production may be an alternative to more severe consequences of genetic translocations in different organ systems. The wide variability of viruses could easily be accounted for by the wide variability of genetic material. Viruses may be a mechanism for managing irritation as an alternative to cancer. Thus, virus "infections" that appear to be highly psychosomatic at times (e.g., the common cold) may be a cellular technique to manage emotional irritation that has been transposed into noxious chemicals (adrenaline, stomach acidity, etc.). Everyone may have body

*Laidlow, P. D., 1938.
**Andrewes, C. H., 1957.

organ (somatic) translocations, but not everyone gets cancer as a result of irritation. We do all suffer from "viral infections."

I am not saying that viruses cannot be communicated. Once formed, they can infect and stimulate others of a similar genetic persuasion—man to man, dog to dog, plant to plant—to replicate the original virus.

Whether viruses are submicroscopic organisms or whether they are a by-product of the cells' defense against a translocated gene, viruses are irritants; and they are carcinogens to some. The fact that viruses can exist for decades without sustenance tends to support the idea that they are a unique nonliving entity. They do not reproduce themselves; they get the cells to do it for them.

If cancer is a reaction to irritation, then one man's virus may be another man's trigger mechanism for cancer. We know that stress affects the immune system, which determines our receptivity to all infection. Under certain types of stress we are far more vulnerable to colds and other diseases. What sets up the predisposition? Genetics and virology have not answered this question.

If viruses are as virulent as many assume, it seems likely that one or another virus would have claimed us and all other life forms on this earth before now. The body's ability to form antigen and antibody defenses apparently is what has saved us.

Having listened to patients explain how they suffer from frequent bouts with rhinoviruses, the "common cold," it greatly interested me that many of them could not recollect when they had had contact with people with colds. They did usually report suffering from anxiety and/or depression. The more stress, the greater the likelihood of falling victim to a cold.

A number of variables must be taken into consideration here. The immune system is less efficient under emotional stress; the cold sufferer may have been in contact with unknown carriers; and perhaps, we produce our own viruses under the right conditions.

A number of viruses seem to be seasonal. Polio was the dread of summer for years; New Year's brings a wave of cold infections; influenza seems to prefer January.

Most virologists seem to agree that no specific season or weather conditions are relevant to the common cold. Chilling does not seem to be a major factor; rainfall and wind seem to be immaterial; but sudden seasonal changes in the weather do appear to be important.

Mental health professionals have long observed that not just colds seem to result from seasonal climatic changes. Ulcers and colitis, which are certainly not viral, appear to be even more difficult to tolerate and manage at these times, and we are confident that they are psychosomatic disorders.

Seasonal changes in climate may not be an adequate physical or chemical explanation for bodily changes, but this climatic phenomenon does create shifts in routine and patterns that can be superficially slight but provide sufficient degrees of emotional irritation for some individuals. This irritation may or may not be noticed at the time, but it may trigger the discharge of the translocated gene.

Another significant fact is that the irritation of receiving several innoculations at the same time seems to increase the risk of getting a cold. A study was done at Great Lakes Naval Training Station where recruits received many vaccinations at one time. The instructors did not. The "boots" frequently got colds, while the instructors exposed to the same viruses did not. The study assumed this was due to physiological stress from the chemical compounds injected into the new sailors. What was ignored was the anxiety and fears to which rigorous military training subjects the inductees. I believe that if adequate studies were done on college or graduate students around the time of final exams, the frequency of colds would be shown to correlate.

It is common, as well as scientific, knowledge that children's colds are more virulent and communicable than adults'. Is it possible that the rate of growth in children has something to do with this? After infancy, growth slows down but still remains rapid up to adulthood. This rapid reproduction of cells through mitosis may be characterized by numerous translocations in some children. If their defense against the somatic misplaced nucleic acids is the production of viruses, is it possible that they would then be emitting far greater concentrations of viruses? This could account for the long-observed phenomenon of children's colds being far more infectious than adults'.

After millions of dollars, thousands of man hours, and even discovering the viruses involved, we still have no cure for the common cold. Perhaps the mechanisms are more internal than previously assumed. We have been looking at issues either from the outside in or the inside out. Is it possible that, like cancer research, we have been ignoring the whole person?

It is possible that the spontaneous generation of viruses is one form of defense against cancer by expelling misplaced nucleic acid before it can trigger cancerous reactions.

The generation of viruses in response to environmental influence was first demonstrated by André Wolf right after World War II. These genetic phenomena are easier to study in bacteria than in more advanced organisms. Ptashne, Johnson, and Pabo* have recently demonstrated that E. Coli bacteria generate viruses if exposed to ultraviolet radiation. According to noted British virologist C. H. Andrewes,** the body is known to produce legions of viruses that cause no symptoms at all in humans; illness does not have to be a result of spontaneous generation of viruses. These viruses may be merely the outcome of the cells' natural defense against translocated genetic material. Susceptibility to viral infections and, perhaps, the spontaneous generation of viruses may indicate, to some extent, an unusually high degree of sensitivity to irritation.

*Ptashne, M., Johnson, A., and Pabo, C., 1982.
**Andrewes, C. H., 1957.

As previously stated, antibodies and antigens have little effect upon viruses once they are within a cell. But the spread of viruses may be halted in an entirely different way: interferon. For many years we have known that an infection by one virus (cowpox) may protect cells from other viruses (smallpox) through a process called interference. Interferon appears to be the modulator of this process. It is a low molecular weight protein that is made within the cells. It can work on a virus where antibodies cannot. Virus damage or misplaced nucleic acid stimulates the cell to produce interferon. It works against viruses of different families, not just the stimulator. It appears to be species specific in that one animal type of interferon will not work in other animals. It prevents the spread of viruses from one cell to the next, containing the virus within the original cell.

Until now there has been no dramatic success in treating cancer with interferon. In fact, if interferon causes the containment of a virus in the individual cells, it may actually trigger or spread cancer in the organism. Anything that would prevent the expulsion of misplaced nucleic acid may in actuality deprive the cell of a defense against evolving into a cancerous unit.

Recently researchers at the National Cancer Institute in Washington, D.C., reported a study that casts grave doubts upon the use of interferon in treating cancer.* In laboratory experiments, Ewing sarcoma, a bone cancer usually afflicting children, "invaded healthy" cells by an increase of three, seventeen, and twenty-two times the normal rate, depending upon which of the three basic forms of interferon was used. The research leader admitted that this was an unexpected result. The study states: "Clearly, the relative importance of the effects of interferon on the tumor and the (patient) must be assessed for each type of tumor."*

Viruses do cause cancer in subhumans. When administered in

---

*Berger, S. L., 1981.

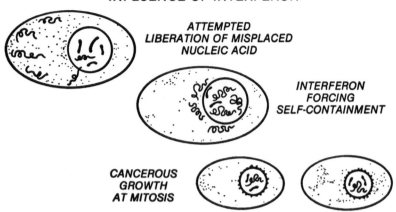

INFLUENCE OF INTERFERON

ATTEMPTED
LIBERATION OF MISPLACED
NUCLEIC ACID

INTERFERON
FORCING
SELF-CONTAINMENT

CANCEROUS
GROWTH
AT MITOSIS

conjunction with other carcinogens, the effects are frequently explosive. In 1909, Francis Peyton Rous found that viruses cause a sarcoma, a malignant connective-tissue tumor, in fowl. Rous's sarcoma has been intensively studied ever since.

And we have all heard of the use of white mice, rats, etc., to study pervasive cancers as well as tumors.

It is significant that these viruses that cause cancer in rats and mice do not cause it in humans. So why is it that the scientific community continues to study the cancer-causing viruses of the subhumans to seek answers for human cancer? Viruses most frequently have very different effects across species. The mumps virus is related to the dog distemper virus, the Coxsachi virus in man causes hoof-and-mouth disease in cattle.

Laboratory research has also ignored the psychology of chickens, mice, and rats. If my basic premise is correct, that irritation is a necessary component of the causation of cancer, then the degree of sensitivity to irritation will make one species far more susceptible to cancer than another. As we go down the phylogenetic ladder, the hypersensitivity of subhumans is a survival mechanism. Watch a rat in action sometime. All the observable senses are far keener than man's. Touch, taste, smell, hearing, sight are all honed to a razor's edge. Dogs have a sense of smell estimated to be one hundred times as keen as humans'. Observe the startle reaction of a group of chickens. They jump out of their feathers far more often than we jump out of our skins. They are most sensitive to both chemical and physical irritants, or stimuli if you prefer. If a human even approached this degree of sensitivity, he would be locked up in a mental institution.

All of this makes me believe that cancer-related experiments on such animals are close to irrelevant in terms of human studies. All sorts of carcinogens cause mice to develop tumors. Viruses, which can be considered irritants, also cause such reactions. Science has not just been comparing apples to oranges, but apples to elephants. An example may help clarify this vitally important issue. Simian virus 40, which has cross-species effects that support this aspect of my theory, was found in batches of polio vaccine in which it was long undetected because it does not produce changes in rhesus monkey cultures used for making the vaccines. In man, it produced no harmful effects that we know of. But if hamsters are injected with simian virus 40, tumors are produced.

In summary, viruses can serve as carcinogens. But more important, the cell quite possibly produces noxious viruses as well as apparently harmless ones as a means of dealing with the misplaced nucleic acids of genetic translocations. If these nucleic acids cannot be expelled, perhaps because of the generation of interferon, they may, particularly in conjunction with other carcinogens, trigger a cancerous reaction.

But if we look only to carcinogens, or viruses, or genetics, or psychology for the cause of cancer, we will get nowhere. They are *all* related to the cause of cancer.

5

Cancer, a
Learned Response

She is so quiet and shy.
He talks all the time and reveals everything.
My husband accuses me of everything he is guilty of.
My wife is a space cadet. She flakes out all the time reading
romance novels.
He gets violent.
She is promiscuous.
He's an alcoholic.
She is eating herself into an early grave.
He's a pathological liar.
She can't face facts.
He's cheap.
She can't hold onto a dime.
He jogs seven miles a day.
She never moves a muscle.
He's insecure.
She's grandiose.

WE ALL HAVE DEFENSES. Some are so obvious to others that
we think of them as problems. Some are so subtle that we accept
them as personality or character traits.

A defense is a learned pattern of behavior that enables the individual to ward off certain noxious stimuli in the environment. A defense is a survival mechanism; in this sense, it is a good and necessary thing.

Freud at first believed that a person who is subjected to traumatic events in infancy and early childhood suffers in later life from the residual feelings that surrounded the original event. The facts or ideas that could describe the trauma get repressed in the unconscious. But feelings cannot be repressed and, instead, are stored within the body systems. They remain there for an individual's entire life and cause symptoms that at best are an inconvenience and at worst can result in death. The basic orientation of Freudian analysis was to reunite these repressed ideas with the "free-floating" feelings in the body. The use of interpretation within the therapeutic relationship was to be the medium for this reunion.

But what Freud actually found was that connecting the feeling and the idea did little to change the symptoms or the defenses. So he adopted other methods of treatment (working through) when he discovered that the ghosts haunting the body could not be laid to rest by the mere presentation of an explanation of their existence. Telling someone that he does not like women because his mother was rotten to him does not seem to get the patient to give up women-hating.

For our purpose, a defense is a learned pattern of behavior that permits survival of the organism. It is an excellent adaptation in early life to a truly terrible set of circumstances. Usually it is an adaptation to repeated exposure to negative stimuli or irritants. Soldiers, for example, do not usually become shell shocked from one horrible experience. This is true for babies, as well. An isolated incident will rarely cause the child to learn to adapt to a negative set of circumstances. Learning at almost all stages requires repetition. One does not start off playing the piano like Rubinstein.

One traumatic event as the cause of great suffering makes for entertaining reading in novels and for interesting television shows and movies. But in real life if the noxious stimuli were infrequent and short-lived, there will have been insufficient conditioning to establish permanent defenses.

What makes a psychological defense a problem in adulthood is that the infantile learning no longer fits the circumstances. The maintenance of what is originally learned is a part of the human condition. It is hard for us to break old habits because it is hard to abandon patterns of behavior learned in infancy and childhood. In order to continue to use our primary learned defenses, we may even have to distort how we view reality. When this becomes an extreme system, the person's defenses are considered to be insane. In milder instances, the distortion of reality to maintain the learned defense is far more subtle. Either way, the defensive patterns are nothing more than misapplied and misplaced conditioned responses. The original stimulus is not there, so we fabricate it through this distortion of reality. Pathological defenses are again based upon humans doing what is familiar, not what is best.

Peter was an eight-year-old who appeared to be a typical suburban schoolboy. He had two adolescent sisters who were all wrapped up in their equally adolescent boyfriends. His father was an engineer employed by a large defense-related industry. His mother was a past PTA president and a member of her church's women's organization.

Peter's room was decorated with a basketball, catcher's mitt, model airplanes, and pictures of athletic stars on his walls. He had a few friends, but he usually had to call them if he wanted to play with them. He was not close to any of them. His father had tried to interest him in model building, but Peter preferred his obsessional pursuit of fan material from baseball heroes.

Peter was a quiet boy who seemed withdrawn and somewhat depressed. He was uncomfortable with intimacy on any level. His worship of baseball stars was a defense against involvement with other people.

Peter's mother invited a neighbor and her son to lunch because of her concern about Peter's lack of social contact. As the two boys began to play electronic games together, Peter became more and more disagreeable. He chose games that only one person could play at a time, and he made sure that he picked games that he was an expert at. His average playing time was ten minutes a turn. His friend, who had never played these games before, had little success and usually finished his turn in one or two minutes.

Peter would then resume his demonstration of expertise. At first, the friend was fascinated watching him, and he asked questions in order to learn the technique; but Peter became obviously annoyed by questions and interruptions. Before long, the other child wanted to leave.

This was not the first time this kind of thing had happened, and Peter saw it as another justification of his withdrawal and self-containment. This boy, like all the others, did not like him. After all, he had shared his games with him and was still rejected. The next time Peter's mother suggested having a friend over, he ignored her. The repetition and maintenance of the defense was complete.

Peter's defense of withdrawal and self-containment was a survival mechanism from earliest infancy. His mother had not been able to relate to the boy she thought she had always wanted. When the infant Peter sensed her hostile feelings, he attempted to turn them off, with both his body and mind storing the negative stimulation. Because his mother did not like him, Peter generalized that other people did not like him either. He was afraid that they were feeling what his mother felt. His defense of withdrawal and self-containment helped kill him. At the age of ten, Peter died of acute leukemia.

Let us look more closely at the process. Defenses are self-propelled, so to speak. Each time a defense works, there is reason to keep it. Then there is reinforcement and validation of its continued use.

Leukemic children usually appear to have always been withdrawn and somewhat depressed.* Frequently the parents share a similar constellation of defenses. Leukemic children also share the common psychological denominator of not being able to accept unconditional love, particularly when hyperirritated. They cannot be soothed or comforted; they seek to maximize their irritations.

All psychosomatic disorders appear to be centered upon the involuntary or autonomic nervous systems. Even disorders of voluntary muscles are more related to the involuntary aspects of these muscles. For instance, posture and muscle tone are not controlled by the area of the brain that controls the voluntary functions of those muscles. We do not have to think about these things normally. But psychosomatic stress can be focused on these muscle groups, resulting in backaches and muscle spasms.

No one consciously says, "Now that I am upset, I am going to overly secrete hydrochloric acid into my stomach so that I can eat away at my stomach lining and develop a peptic ulcer." We learn this unconscious automatic process as a means of defense against more destructive forces in our environment. We learn these things when feelings are blatantly more important than thoughts. We learn our predisposition to psychosomatic disorders in the earliest stages of our lives. The question remains as to what this conditioning is.

In the first three months of life, we have the human being at the greatest degree of vulnerability to stimulation or irritation. He has lost the protection of the womb. He has no means of intelligently processing the stimulation that impinges upon him from the inside as well as the outside. He is the epitome of rawness. There is only one thing that prevents the overwhelming of the

*Greene, W., 1966.

newborn. This is the emotional entropy of the mother-baby fusion. The capacity for entropy is no more learned in the mother and baby than it is in the previous example of hot soup and a spoon. It is just there. The irritations (hunger, gas, noise, smells, etc.) are decreased by this first psychological and biological defense.

The baby, at this point, has very limited physical needs. His cries and body language serve as an alarm system to initiate physical and emotional nurturance from the mother. There are only so many things one can do to meet the relatively simple biological needs of the newborn. The procedures get repeated and repeated. Relatively quickly the mother will learn the language of her newborn. For example, hunger may be communicated by the loudest, most demanding, and prolonged crying of the baby. His body will, at the same time, communicate by a tightening of the stomach, a drawing up of the legs, a red face, and the waving of both arms. He appears to be in pain, and he probably is. As mother learns to understand her newborn's communications, she will inadvertently be rewarding this use of cries and body language through simple conditioning. Thinking is not involved. The baby is reinforced each time he gives the same signal and the mother responds in the same positive way. This learning precedes consciousness as we understand it for the more mature individual. It is on an organic bodily level. Autism is a stage that precedes cognitive learning.

Once these groupings of the baby crying in a certain way and the baby getting rewarded in a certain way are well established, the child is out of the autistic stage. He is well on the important road to learning that there exists an inside and an outside of himself. He is on the road to learning that others exist in this world.

If the mother meets his needs and fuses with him, he is being conditioned into a lifelong proposition of accepting love and caring when he is hyperirritated. If the mother cannot meet his needs adequately, then he is conditioned to hold his irritation in, to be afraid of having others add to it, and to produce an increased level of internal chemical agents, which soothe one area while irritating another. As the stimulus is not being met by a loving outside response, it is directed inward.

In later life, irritating stimuli from the inside and the outside will result in this same response of keeping it in. At the same time, something in the genetic material may be changing ever so slightly. Cancer can thus be viewed as one mechanism for the organism to *process* irritation.

Why do some people get cancer from irritation while others get a peptic ulcer, for example. The answer lies in the history of the conditioning. If the aberrant learning occurred in the autistic stage, the land mines will be there to explode in a later biological regression to infantile growth. If, however, one makes it through the autistic stage with a minimum of genetic translocations, then all subsequent conditioning for self-containment of irritation will fall upon healthy tissue. The hydrochloric acid of the stomach may be overproducing, but if the tissue and cells it attacks are healthy, the irritation will result in an ulcer. If the cells include many genetic translocations, then the risk of one or several of these cells being triggered into infantile growth because of the addition of irritation is there.

However, an individual who develops an ulcer instead of a stomach tumor is not necessarily immune to cancer of the stomach or other organ systems. Having one benign psychosomatic disorder does not, unfortunately, indicate any protection against subsequent cancer.

This brings us to another important issue of conditioning with regard to cancer. Why is it that some organ systems only rarely succumb to this disorder? The medical profession focuses its attention upon the organ systems that can easily become malignant. Only a few academics and research people study what seems to be relatively immune: the voluntary muscles; the nerve cells; and the extreme appendages, the fingers and toes. Red blood cells are also immune, but they have no nuclei. Without a nucleus, the cell cannot reproduce itself through division. Red blood cells come from nucleated cells, which produce them.

I am not saying that cancer of these systems absolutely never occurs. I am saying that almost no one we hear about ever died from a primary site cancer of the biceps, triceps, lower back muscles, etc. The skin, the bone, the connective tissues immediately near them, yes; but the voluntary or striated muscles, very rarely. When this does occur, it is a true horror of pain and discomfort. But it is a relatively infrequent occurrence. This is true because of the following:

When a baby is born, the organs that most clearly can discharge tension and irritation are the voluntary muscles. All the child has to do is move an arm or leg, tighten the stomach, arch his back, and the irritation is dissipated. Organ systems that cannot discharge as readily and are subjected to a large degree of irritation will be far more vulnerable. Their movement is no more relevant to discharging irritation than the movements of breathing and the lungs or peristalsis and the stomach. The more stationary systems will be more vulnerable.

Fingers and toes are *rarely* primary sites of malignancies.* Why? Take another look at the newborn. Fingers and toes clutch and release. The release is frequently a rigid extension of both. It appears as if the baby is trying to get rid of something through this movement. This something is irritation. An older autistic child will shake his entire hand while moving his fingers.

Now we come to one of the most fascinating aspects of this theory. Most of us know of someone who has suffered, and possibly died, from a brain tumor. We know that nerve cells are not capable of even normal division while in the body. People with

*Conversation with Dr. L. Liegner, 1982; conversation with Dr. L. Kaplan, 1983.

spinal cord injuries in which the cord is severed have no chance of recovery. The cells are destroyed and do not regenerate. If the entire cord is not severed, neighboring cells and pathways may assume some functioning with some "recovery." Nerve cells, which will be referred to as neurons from this point on, are "postmitotic"; they do not divide.

Irritation on some level is necessary to trigger cell division. Whether the irritation is the normal high hormonal levels of infancy, injury, or carcinogens, something gets to the nucleus and the genetic material inside it. Neurons have viable nuclei with a full complement of chromosomes. It is their physiological function that prevents them from dividing either normally or malignantly. When an irritant reaches the cell membrane of the neuron, an entire electrochemical system is activated to discharge the irritant and pass it on as an electrochemical signal to the next neuron, all the way to the brain. This function of neurons prevents the nucleus from being irritated enough to cause cell division. If there were enough irritation to overcome the electrochemical functioning of the cell, it would kill it before it could nudge it into division.

Then what of brain or spinal cord tumors? Neuropathologists have told me that it is the supportive cells that become malignant in these tumors. The insulating cells of the sheath can become malignant. More typically it is such cells as the glial (supportive) cells that absorb this irritation and reproduce malignantly.

There remains the issue of neuroblastomas, a malignancy of the neuroblasts. These are the embryological cells that give rise to the neurons. On occasion, they remain as residual embryological tissues after birth. When this happens, they can reproduce as more neuroblasts. Tragically this usually affects children one or two years of age. But these are not cancerous neurons. It is not impossible for a neuron to be malignant. However, no one I spoke to on a professional level who studies these issues had ever seen or heard of such an occurrence.

85

These organ systems are important because of their relative immunity to cancer. They all share the property of being unable to be hyperirritated during autistic-stage development. Thus, they cannot develop genetic translocation as a defense against being overwhelmed by irritation. Voluntary muscles, fingers, and toes discharge immediately through the simpler defense of movement. Neurons discharge or totally shut down in response to hyperirritation. Cells must be vulnerable to hyperirritation to undergo translocation.

Let us return to the matter of conditioning as it affects later cancer. We have seen how cancer can be conditioned inadvertently in our newborns. To understand better some of the subsequent issues in this book with regard to medical and psychological treatment, we must start with the basics of learning theory. Once a defensive pattern has been conditioned, how can we stop or extinguish it?

Several years ago, I was treating a paranoid schizophrenic in a hospital. She explained to me how the powers that be had stolen both her inventions and her writings. Her pen name was Herman Hesse, and she had invented radar during World War II, she said.

Every other therapist she had had contact with had confronted her with the facts that she was Jane Smith from Brooklyn, New York, and had not even been born when World War II took place. And every other therapist had been immediately dismissed by her. When she first came into my office, she reported that there was a plain unmarked car in the lot outside. It was the FBI that was after her.

Patient: They want to kill me rather than ante up for what they stole from me.
Analyst: What was that?
Patient: You won't believe me, either, but I invented radar and wrote some very successful books.
Analyst: You aren't going to tell me anything that would get them after *me*, are you?

Patient: Are you afraid of them, too?

Analyst: Listen, I know how unethical and corrupt any government people can be.

Patient: Okay, then what should we talk about?

Analyst: Hold it a minute. Did you hear anything at the door? [I got up, opened the door, looked up and down the hallway, and sat back down.] No one there, but I could have sworn I heard someone listening to us.

Patient: Are you always so afraid of other people?

Analyst: What do you think?

Patient: I think you are, just like me.

This cemented a relationship that permitted this young, truly brilliant woman to leave the state hospital system. A great deal of additional work ensued, but this first exposure convinced her that I was safe because I was like her. The purpose of her distorted reality was to maintain her feelings of being sufficiently important to be persecuted by government agencies—or anyone. My respecting and actually going along with such defenses made it possible for her not to maintain such an investment in them. Eventually she was to tell me that she was becoming aware of her distortions, but she continued them because they *felt* so good.

This is an important point. We maintain our conditioned responses, which we call defenses, because of the emotional involvement in them. Any attempt at correcting or reversing these defenses through using thought as the medium is a waste of time.

It is also important to remember that the more invested an individual is in her earliest learning, the more likely it is that her parents had a need for her to be a quiet good baby. This means that she would have had to internalize her upsets, impulses, or irritations.

If I had told my patient that the FBI car was really owned by the New York State Office of Mental Health and was used to ferry patients around, in all probability any possibility of successful treatment would have been immediately destroyed. She would have felt misunderstood, and she would have dismissed me as being merely another dumb shrink in the state system.

This type of psychotherapeutic intervention is referred to as a *reflective technique.** It amounts to walking downstream with a patient rather than attempting to walk upstream in the therapeutic river. It gives the patient the opportunity to perceive the analyst as safe enough to reexperience the patient's earlier fusion with him. It thus permits an emotional reeducation.

This important concept of *psychological reflection* requires explanation. We can condition a pigeon to press a lever. After numerous repetitions, he learns that every time he presses the lever he gets another pellet of food. Now, how do we get the pigeon to stop pressing the lever? There are several options. The simplest is merely to cut off the supply of food pellets. Eventually, the pigeon will learn that pecking at the lever means that nothing will happen. This is a long, drawn-out process, with frequent reoccurrences of lever-pressing optimism.

We could also arrange to shock the bird every time he presses the lever. This is a much faster but inefficient mechanism for extinguishing conditioned responses. Again reoccurrences of the previous learning happen in spite of the punishment.

The third option is perhaps the most direct and, for some reason, the least obvious. We can get the pigeon to stop his food-seeking behavior by feeding or satiating the drive motivating the conditioned response. He will not be the least bit interested in pressing the lever as long as he is satiated. But as soon as he is hungry again, he will fall back on the conditioned response to the stimulus of hunger.

The realm of psychopharmacology provides viable examples of the use of reflective techniques. In the case of the hyperactive child, the use of Ritalin or other central nervous system stimu-

*Spotnitz, H., 1969.

lants results in the temporary reduction of hyperactivity. For the most part, the medical descriptions of why and how these drugs work to calm the hyperkinetic child are vaguely summarized by stating that the drugs have a "paradoxical effect."

If psychological reflection is taken into account, the effects of these stimulants upon the hyperactive child may be viewed as a satiation of the motivation of the conditioned response of hyperactivity. This, of course, assumes that hyperkinesis is an emotionally conditioned response. Adding a drug that causes agitation or a hyperactive state to a conditioned response of extremes of movement results in a satiation of the response. Once this satiation occurs, the child is temporarily calm. Reoccurrence of the response follows the wearing off of the drug. The same thing usually happens if we place hyperactive children in a moving car. They will frequently calm down as effectively as if they had been given Ritalin. The car's movement satiates the conditioned response. After the ride, the hyperkinesis returns.

Some fascinating work was done by Stanislas Groff on the experimental use of LSD in the treatment of schizophrenics. LSD-25 is a psychotic mimetic; that is, it causes the individual to experience mental functioning similar to the functioning of a psychotic. Groff administered LSD-25 to psychotic, neurotic, and "normal" groups. The psychotic group manifested rapid but short-lived symptom abatement; the neurotic group showed slight improvement, marked by a rapid return to previous symptoms (conditioned responses); the normal group showed symptoms of psychosis.

This experiment appears to demonstrate that if LSD-25, which acts to mimic psychosis, is added to a preexisting psychotic state, it will temporarily satiate the conditioned responses of psychosis and will extinguish the symptoms temporarily. With the psychoneurotic group, the marginal improvement can be viewed as the effect upon marginal symptoms. With the normal population, the LSD-25 would be oppositional to the mature and adequate conditioned response of this group. Only when the drug was added to preexisting symptoms was there a temporary satiation of the emotional aspects of the conditioned response.

In the paranoid, the conditioned response of grandiosity defends against feelings of being weak and ineffectual. The use of drugs such as Thorazine (phenothiazines in general) makes an individual feel weak and tired. Thus, these drugs can be viewed as attacking the conditioned responses of the paranoid rather than satiating them.

What does all of this have to do with cancer? Reflective psychology can be used as a succinct and precise explanation of why most medical interventions work initially to cause an extinction of the conditioned responses of maximizing irritation and self-destruction that I find in cancer patients. In medical terms, psychological reflection can explain how and why remissions (reduction or eradication of symptoms) occur after medical intervention. It also explains why the conditioned responses (symptoms) of cancer all too frequently reoccur (spontaneous recovery of the conditioned response).

The next chapter discusses these medical issues.

6

Modern Medical
Techniques

BARBARA WAS DIAGNOSED as having breast cancer two years after her divorce. She is thirty-eight years old and has two daughters. She has not been able to find anyone desirable to date. Usually the men she has brief relationships with are not interested in anything permanent.

Barbara has had a malignant tumor removed from her left breast. She also has had eleven lymph nodes in her armpit removed surgically. Her initial emotional torture was hearing that she had cancer, followed immediately by the additional conflict over what type of surgery to have.

"I consulted three different surgeons before I had my lumpectomy. The first one wanted to do a mastectomy. The second recommended taking what he saw as the safest route: a radical mastectomy. The last one I saw recommended the lumpectomy. He showed me studies that seemed to prove that, if the lump is small enough, it is as successful as the more severe disfiguring procedures.

"After the operation, the oncologists [cancer specialists] began on me. I went to seven of them for opinions. I got seven different recommendations. They all took the time to explain what the recommendations were based on. Most recommended radiation and chemotherapy in close proximity. Some said I should have received radiation during surgery. Others said chemo should have been started sooner. The radiologists all made it clear that neighboring tissue could be made cancerous as they burned the already-affected tissues. They said that they were more precise and exact than ever before, but they all explained that there were risks.

"When it came to chemotherapy the divergence of opinion was unbelievable! Seven doctors told me to do seven different things. Most included the same drugs but added or subtracted from the list. I don't know what they based their choices on. Some wanted to knock the cancer out with a powerful sudden onslaught. Others said if we did that, we would be very limited in future treatment. These guys recommended that I start gently or moderately so if the cancer came back or spread, there would be more options.

"Which makes more sense to you? I don't know. Both arguments seemed very logical to me. But what do I know? I'm not a doctor. Maybe I was wrong in researching the whole thing so thoroughly. Anyway, what it literally came down to was that I had to pick my own poison! Everyone of them explained that chemotherapy was based on poisoning and killing all the really rapidly reproducing cells in my body. This would mean the cancer cells, too, of course.

"What finally happened was that I went with a doctor who recommended a moderate approach. That seemed less scary to me, but to be honest, I still don't have any idea which makes more sense. Dr. Schwartz was someone I could relate to. He listened and seemed to be genuinely concerned. I know this is weird, but I had similar feelings about the doctor who delivered my babies. I trusted these men; something was different about them. Another doctor said that I might still have a chance of surviving if I listened to him. He scared me so much, I just about ran out of the office. Schwartz is the nicest and most reasonable, even though I still don't know how to reason about any of this. He told me that I should talk to someone like you. He said there is so much we don't understand about cancer that maybe stress and other feelings have something to do with it.

"Dr. Schwartz told me that in most cases breast cancer is systemic, that was his word. I guess it means they spread a lot. He said that by the time a lump is large enough to be felt malignant cells have been around for two to five years. They most likely have been spread throughout the body and can cause other tumors—you know, metastasize. He said a lot goes into the fight against this spreading. Dr. Schwartz believes feelings have a lot to do with all this. He said he's seen enough women with similar life histories to question the psychology of this part of it. His recommendation seemed to mean he cared and that you would have the time to handle the emotional parts of it. But he always sat and talked with me for some time.

"When I got really scared, he told me that he would be my doctor no matter what. Once in a while he put a hand on my shoulder as I left his office. It always made me feel warm and calm all over. The fact that Michael Schwartz, M.D., is a gorgeous hunk does not hurt in the least either!"

Whatever the organ systems involved or diagnosed as the primary site, the surgical procedures for treating cancer amount to basically the same thing. The earlier the diagnosis and the more localized the malignancy, the smaller the amount of the body that is cut out. Surgery is a highly sophisticated medical specialty. Fortunately, new trends in surgery cause less disfigurement than in the past. For example, until recently almost everyone with colon cancer had a colostomy. Today, only about one patient in seven requires it. Limb cancer does not necessarily result in amputation today. Instead, when possible, just the cancerous part is cut away, and radiation is applied.

But even if less severe than it used to be, cancer surgery is usually nothing more than cutting out parts of the body.

Radiation therapy is based upon exposing the cancerous, or

likely to be cancerous, tissues to the burning effects of radioactive agents. These may be generated by technical machinery or isotopes. Radioactive tubes or capsules may be placed upon the body for short periods of time. This is practical only if the cancer is relatively close to the surface. For more deeply buried cancer, the capsules or tubes may be surgically implanted. After a period of usually a couple of days, they must be removed before too much healthy tissue is destroyed. Techniques for determining dosage and administration are highly sophisticated. They are getting progressively more and more sophisticated in the attempt to limit the risk of inducing subsequent cancer and destroying neighboring tissue.

Implant radiation is usually preferable to avoid damaging neighboring cells. The surgeon implants radioactive pellets or weaves a radioactive thread in or around a tumor. Pellets and threads have been used for gynecological, lung, pancreatic, head, and neck cancer with good results. Intraoperative radiation allows healthy organs to be moved out of the way to allow exact placement of the radioactive agent during surgery. Up to four times the dosage can be given intraoperatively as opposed to traditional therapy from the outside.

The type of radiation is likely to change in the near future. Neutron radiation is being investigated by the National Cancer Institute as a more efficient, lower energy, and higher kill ratio agent than the traditional X-ray radiation.

However, all that this technology boils down to is burning cancerous tissue out of existence.

Chemotherapies are based upon the property that all cancer has in common: a rapid and apparently random reproduction of affected cells. Most cancers have different periods or cycles of growth. The idea is to have a regimen of poison available that will kill rapidly reproducing cells in the time cycles of the cancers. Normally, four or five drugs will be utilized to make sure that one is present to intercept the cancerous reproduction along this time continuum. If one chemical does not do the cancer in, the next cycle will be covered by the next chemical.

In recent years, we have progressed amazingly in the pharmacological treatment of cancer. However, chemotherapies still have the obvious problem that the most effective anticancer drugs (poisons) have the worst side effects. Techniques are being devised to test which drugs the patient's cancer cells will respond to. Dosages are being experimented with in terms of lower, but more frequent, exposure. Research is underway to try to find a monoclonal antibody that will search out and destroy malignant growth. It would be the biological equivalent of a smart bomb.

But at this time, any agent entering the body to kill rapidly reproducing cells will kill healthy rapidly reproducing cells as well as cancerous ones. Thus, hair loss is a common side effect, as are nausea and diarrhea. They can be exceedingly uncomfortable at times.

Standard procedures for chemotherapies for cancer rest on the basic premise of poisoning the cancer cells.

This leaves us with the somewhat disconcerting fact that standard modern cancer treatment is based upon cutting, burning, and poisoning. Granted that these procedures are being used with the utmost care in administration in order to limit the damage to neighboring healthy tissue. But they still add up to cutting, burning, and poisoning, and they all have uncomfortable or even painful side effects as other tissue besides that which is cancerous gets sacrificed.

In biological terms, the side effects of the standard medical procedures are obviously very negative. But psychologically they are wonderful! In fact, they are an important cause of the success of these medical techniques. The practitioner will say that the removal of the cancerous cells is the critical issue. To a great degree this is probably true. But the negative side effects may be as important as, if not more important than, the excising through cutting, burning, and poisoning.

Now, we can at least partially integrate the discussion of conditioning and psychological reflection with popular medical treatment.

Let us go back to our pigeon. Remember that we have several options to get him to stop pressing the lever in order to get a food pellet. If we stop supplying the pellets, eventually he will stop pecking, although he will still keep giving it an occasional optimistic try.

If we shock him each time he presses the lever, he will soon stop. But again he will relatively quickly try to sneak a peck if he is hungry enough.

However, if we feed him to his limit (that is, satiate his hunger drive), the motivation for food-seeking behavior is suspended. When he again experiences hunger, he will press the lever unless we feed him again. This satiation of the drive of the conditioned response is the basic psychodynamic issue of medical treatment for cancer.

Since cancer may be viewed as a conditioned response of hypersensitivity in the face of irritation, it is the fulfillment of the infantile conditioning for destruction through self-containment. What then are we doing when we cut, burn, or poison cancer patients? We are, in effect, satiating the preexisting conditioned response. We are adding so much insult to injury that the initial injury gets suspended.

First, we scare the patients to the extreme degree—we tell them they have cancer. This fear is an aid psychologically in that it facilitates the necessary emotional regression.

Then, in a controlled way, we inflict enough discomfort and pain with our techniques to overwhelm the system. We extinguish the conditioned response.

Medical people call this the process of remission. The cancer has been fed its virgin and can slink back into its cave, at least until it is hungry again. As long as the cancer is being psychologically reflected by medical techniques, the disorder is usually going to at least slow down. The pigeon (unconscious dynamics) has been fed. The lever goes unpressed until the need for food (self-destruction) arises. The hypersensitivity that was originally conditioned is being thoroughly overwhelmed by the administration of enormous amounts of irritation. The need to self-destruct is being buried under the destruction of healthy and cancerous cells. The food is cutting, burning, or poisoning.

A rather rare medical occurrence was reported to me by a physician. A fifty-two-year-old man suffered a heart attack upon hearing that he had a large colon cancer that required surgery. The heart attack precluded the colon operation. Three months later, tests of all kinds could find no trace of colon cancer. Two years later, there was still no sign of cancer. What had happened? The physician said that he believed that healing enzymes were produced by the body in response to the heart attack. In his opinion, this cured the cancer.

I believe the conditioned response of self-destruction was satiated by the immediate fear of annihilation from the heart attack. A serious heart attack is terrifying. It adds an overwhelming irritation. The pigeon has now been fed. The self-destructive patient now didn't *need* the irritation of cancer.

Some patients may, through treatment, have enough irritation added to the infantile hypersensitivity to irritation to keep them well fed for a lifetime. The cancer seems gone. (Cure is a word most medical people are reticent to use in regard to this disorder for cancer may rear its ugly head again years later. Thus, a more appealing way to put it is that *the disease is in remission.*)

Others may need periodic feedings to satiate the self-destructive drives. Eventually they cannot be fed anymore, for the feeding may in itself be lethal. The patient dies, usually not from the direct effects of the cancer but from its destructive side effects. Pneumonia, other infections, cardiac problems, and a general wasting away are typically the causes of death.

Medical procedures are necessary. The suffering they cause

may, however, be as important as the attempt to excise cancer directly. Too often, subsequent tumors or reoccurrences appear, and the medical practitioner must sadly admit that some cells may have gotten away from the surgeon's knife, the radiotherapist's burns, or the chemotherapist's poisons.

It is also possible that any individual with translocations in one organ system will have them in others. In advanced metastasized cancer, it seems almost as if the cancer is trying to get out of the body. Now fingers and toes can become secondary sites.

Those schizophrenic children who shake their hands and wiggle their fingers may be trying to rid themselves of something to which we have been blind: *Cancer is the body's reaction to any and all irritation severe or habitual enough to reach the translocated genetic material.*

7

Carcinogens: Tangible and Intangible

FOR YEARS THERE HAVE BEEN media scares that make it seem as if *everything* is carcinogenic. One Thanksgiving, it was cranberry sauce. Cigarettes, saccharin, the sun, X rays, microwaves, air pollution, water pollution, red meat, nitrous amines, the pill, etc., have all been portrayed as lethal.

To point up the need to keep things in perspective, two research scientists did a tongue-in-cheek experiment on albino white rats. They implanted quarters and dimes in the rats' abdomens. Sure enough, almost every rat subjected to these implants developed cancer somewhere in the abdomen and died. The researchers hypothesized that even close proximity to this highly toxic pollutant could be a risk and suggested that it should be removed from the environment. With almost reckless disregard for their own safety, they asked that everyone in the country send their quarters and dimes, preferably in rolls, to them. They would brave the danger in order to help their countrymen avoid the probability of getting abdominal cancer and succumbing like the rats!

Americans are obsessed with chemical and physical carcinogens. The latest, and perhaps most popular, area of carcinogen concern centers on nutrition. This is a tangible over which we have some control.

The scientific investigation of the nutritional aspects of cancer received support in 1980 when the National Cancer Institute began to study diet and cancer. As a result of the investigation, the institute recommended a 30 to 40 percent reduction in consumption of saturated and unsaturated fats and the inclusion of grain, fruits, and vegetables in our daily diet. Citrus fruits and carotene were especially emphasized. It was also recommended that alcohol be consumed only in moderation. (For years physicians have observed that alcoholics were more likely than other people to suffer from digestive-tract cancer.) Smoked, cured, or pickled foods were singled out as high risk additions to diet, and it was pointed out that barbecuing or other high temperature cooking appears to form carcinogens in food. A lot of public attention is now being focused on free-radical ions as carcinogens. These are liberated and charged chemical elements from food that some believe serve as a trigger mechanism for cancer.

The combination of irritants being consumed at the same time certainly would seem to increase the risk of cancer. Thus, if you smoke and drink at the same time, the esophagus, respiratory tract, and the larynx are all being doubly battered. Nonsmoking alcoholics are more likely to get just colon or rectal cancer.

It is also necessary to consider the volume of food consumed. People who overeat are obviously putting a greater strain on the digestive system. It is worth noting that in those supposedly healthier countries where low amounts of fat and red meat are consumed, low amounts of food in general are consumed.

What are we to believe? It is true that there is an increased risk of breast and colon cancer in countries where large amounts of red meat and fat in general are consumed. However, in these same countries, air and water pollution levels are higher, and these industrialized nations seem to function with a different mental set than underdeveloped nations. In any event, in nations where meat is a luxury and being a vegetarian is a necessity, not a choice, the contamination from other carcinogens, tangible and intangible, may also be far less than ours.

We do know that consuming pesticides and other industrial pollutants through our food is certainly irritating to our systems. What we do not know is whether eliminating free-radical ion foods; meats and fats; processed foods; smoked, cured, and pickled foods; barbecued food; saccharin; alcohol; etc., will be shown to lower the frequency of cancer in humans.*

Many people are turning to vitamin supplements as a means of cancer prevention, but what research has been done in the field has been done mainly with animals and is inconclusive. In addition, megadoses of vitamins may actually be harmful, and it is wiser to concentrate on a well-balanced diet.

But most important, manipulating our diets and vitamin intake is something within our control. It makes us feel that we have some power over our lives. Actually, in the face of cancer, we may be creating a totem.

Some people can eat fatty barbecued hamburgers, pickles, and potato chips; drink beer; and smoke cigarettes while working in a polluted city on a sunny day and still not get cancer. It is true that they may succumb to something else before cancer can develop, but some will live to an old age while immersed in carcinogens. The puzzling questions for researchers in this field *can* be answered by looking at the *intangible* (emotional and life event) carcinogens.

These intangibles are intangible only because we choose to ignore what we cannot observe and understand simply and directly. The major carcinogen for all of us is an aberrant processing of all irritants. The body may be under attack from all sorts of stimuli. If we have been conditioned into a precancerous personality, we are going to get cancer. If we have not, the risks are far

*Ames, B., 1983.

less but are still there since no one can be raised without any genetic translocations. But the fewer and less intense their occurrence, the less likely that the tangible carcinogens will fall on target. The chemicals our bodies produce will have fewer target sites, also.

Through experimental work done with biofeedback,* we have been able to demonstrate that previously believed psychologically inaccessible body functions can be conditioned. We can *learn* to increase or decrease things such as heart rate, blood pressure, etc. We thus have a scientific basis for believing that we can learn to produce or not produce internal carcinogens such as adrenaline or hydrochloric acid. Our defense systems can, perhaps, be trained to handle the isolated explosion adequately.

Recently, Adler and Cohen of the University of Rochester conditioned mice to suppress their own immune systems. The research was confirmed at two other laboratories. It is safe to assume that this is only the beginning of what we can learn to do.

The precancerous personality is the ultimate carcinogen. What creates this personality? As genetic translocations are being laid down due to hyperirritation of the newborn, certain psychological conditioning is taking place at the same time. One cannot occur without the other. The first stage of extrauterine life is the significant-age category biologically because of rapid mitotic growth like none other in life except, perhaps, with cancer.

It is important to note that hormone levels in many malignant tumors are the same as in an infant.** In a normal adult lung there is no ACTH (a growth hormone). In a cancerous adult lung ACTH is at the same level as in a newborn baby's lung. This tends to add credence to the beginning of cancer being in the autistic stage. It also suggests that cancer is in some ways a biological return to this stage of life.

*Fuller, G. D., 1978.
**Sugano, H., and Sasano, N., 1980.

Psychologically, the baby is vulnerable to translocations because of a lack of adequate emotional defenses in the face of irritations of all kinds. The precancerous personality has a need to maximize irritations to levels similar to that experienced in infancy. Such an individual will always make a mountain out of a molehill. On top of this need to make the worst rather than the best of any situation, he will have a self-contained system of processing this hyperirritation. Not only is such a person obsessive about how terrible things are, but events in life that he has no control over fit right into his need to repeat infantile hyperirritation. Remember: We do and even feel and think that which is familiar, not that which is best for us.

Patient: Tomorrow I am going on vacation. After all these plans to go to Europe to ski, we are finally having snow forecast in New England. I knew this would happen.

Analyst: Can you change your plans?

Patient: No, we sent in the money, and the kids really want to go. Tonight, it's supposed to start snowing, and I don't know if we will even take off as planned. Have you ever spent hours in an airport waiting for the weather to clear? How about with three kids? It drives me crazy. I begin to feel sick to my stomach and usually get a headache. The airlines don't care. But then I guess I'm happy they aren't taking off in bad weather. The food they serve usually stinks. My wife always manages to get a cold just before we leave, and then I get it when we are in the middle of the vacation. At least snow conditions are always good in the French Alps, but the skiing is not the least bit challenging compared to Colorado or Jackson Hole, Wyoming.

Analyst: Why don't you just stay home and relax for two weeks?

Patient: Are you kidding? My house is an asylum!

Analyst: Are you saying it doesn't matter what the circum-

stances are, you still feel irritated by just about everything?

Patient: I guess that's what I'm saying. And I can't complain to
June, anymore. She tells me to knock it off, that she
can't stand it. She can't change the weather anyway!

For this patient, life was a continuum of upsets and irritations.
Getting caught in traffic was a disaster. Business, which he was
a spectacular success at, was a never-ending supply of emotional
irritation. Something could always go wrong. Success was never
enough, nor did it provide security and confidence. The balloon
could always pop.

This kind of person will always twist his insides over what
could go wrong, not just what does go wrong. He is two steps
ahead of each anticipated catastrophe. His endocrine system is in
a constant state of hyperdrive. But, worst of all is his apparent
lack of adequate psychological defenses.

The precancerous individual, lacking the emotional entropy
that should have been taught in infancy, will be unable to fuse
with anyone else as a means of dissipating irritation. He will most
likely be able to experience intimacy only when he is caring for
someone else. This is safe. To be loved and cared for, however,
results in emotional discomfort, an uneasiness that is easily
detected. The precancerous individual cannot conceal it. Most of
the time he rebuffs caring with bodily reactions of blushing,
stiffness, and an obvious need to push away. It is easy for a person
attempting to soothe a precancerous individual to feel rejected
and angered by his reactions.

Let me give an example. Two men have had a horrendous day
at work. Upon arriving home, the first one says, "Come over here,
honey. I need a hug. Today was rotten in the office. Kids, what
went on in school? Just sit for a minute and talk to me about it."
The precancerous individual enters his home saying, "Just keep
the kids away from me for a while. I had a rotten day, and I don't

want to be with anyone. Let me have an hour or so alone watching the game, and I'll settle down. Just keep them quiet!"

If at the same time he attempts to soothe his irritation with external carcinogens, the problem is intensified. He may be a chronic cigarette smoker and/or alcohol abuser. He may also have a "thing" for one type of food that makes him feel better (a lot of depressed people are chocolate addicts), and any one nutrient in great and habitual excess may become a carcinogen.

He may also soothe his emotional upsets through retreating into isolated activities. At the peak of irritation, absorption with woodworking, needlepoint, books, music, etc., may again be indicative of the precancerous individual's self-contained entropic system.

Mood swings are also a clear symptom. The ability to express rage is no more than an indicator that such an individual is hyperirritated. He will hold onto his anger even after a genuine apology. Righteous indignation has its roots in the precancerous conditioning of the autistic stage.

On the other hand, this individual may be depressed a great deal of the time and never express rage. He may be candy coated as compensation for the anger and irritation he holds inside. The important issue is his inability to accept being loved. Significantly the John Wayne or macho image comes to mind. Men like this would not cry for their mothers in the face of overwhelming irritation. Even the threat of annihilation would not cause them to allow fusion to occur.

Tough is one precancerous characteristic, distance is another. In our society, men can still more easily resort to both. Women are usually still confined to the latter. The precancerous personality will permit friendships as long as they are not very intimate. He will allow a friendship in which the other individual receives. He is an excellent giver. This serves as a defense against the discomfort of receiving. Usually his social adaptation is somewhat extreme. He may join many groups, or he may be reclusive and withdrawn. In either event, the purpose is to resist intimacy and loving.

The fear of closeness stems from the residual fears of events in the autistic stage. When the baby was already irritated, he did not need a mother whose irritation would overwhelm him. Throughout life, the precancerous individual resists truly close contact with the irritating mother. This becomes generalized to the world at large as well as to significant others: a spouse, siblings, children, and friends.

This early conditioning has other effects that are often overlooked. The precancerous personality will have instances of elevated functioning of the senses. Many cancer patients have told me that they see, hear, and smell things before others do. At times they begin to doubt their own perceptions. This is not paranoia but rather a conditioned hypersensitivity in one or all sensory systems. This may be an asset in war, but it can have serious consequences any other time. One patient reported seeing a dozen deer in the forest when his camping partners saw only the one on the road. Imagine his consternation when he even pointed them out and no one else could see them! One patient reported that she could smell things long before other people. She soon learned not to mention it. The question "Did you hear that?" quickly gets surpressed so that others will not think one is hallucinating.

Touch and taste can also be more sensitive. Reactions bordering on allergies or allergies themselves are not uncommon. Wool or terrycloth may be unbearable. The appreciation of spicy foods or the total avoidance of it are also part of this diagnosis.

But most obvious of the psychological symptoms of the precancerous personality is the ultimate autistic residual, the drifting away, the "spaciness." When overwhelmed, the precancerous individual will frequently exercise this option. He will show no significant signs of schizophrenia, but he can retreat into his own inner space totally. Teenagers call such people "space cadets." Precancerous individuals move in and out of this state, which

106

seems to be a refuge for them. If they are impinged upon, they will be at least aggravated if not totally enraged.

Any survey of the causes of cancer that does not include the assessment of autistic residuals ignores the central carcinogen in our lives.

The questions asked in chapter 1 can now all be answered.

Why do divorced or widowed women get breast and cervical cancer more frequently than married women? Because of an abrupt disruption of their relationship, their emotional entropy. A terrible relationship is better than none at all. Even if the marriage was very bad, it could have served to syphon off some irritation. With the end of a sexual relationship, the sexual organ systems will be the focus of—and undischarged—irritation.

If you have lost a parent before the age of seven, your risk of cancer increases because emotional entropy was abruptly ended.

Other situations in life correlate to cancer. A combat soldier exposed to annihilation goes through severe emotional regressions. As his comrades are killed, emotionally entropic relationships are abruptly ended. Add a potent external chemical carcinogen coincidental with this return to early emotionality, and cancer could be a likely outcome.

The fact that dioxin, as in Agent Orange, can cause translocations in the sperm of veterans exposed to it is confirmed by the high incidence of birth defects in their children. If the chemical irritated the body cells, the veteran faces cancer. If it focused on the spermatozoa, the veteran's children pay the price of the translocations.

It is not uncommon for someone to develop cancer while serving a jail term. The loss of a child is also a significant trigger. Again, we have abrupt endings of emotional entropic systems.

The study in southern California and Utah of the Mormons' apparent relative immunity to cancer in the face of chemical and physical carcinogens concluded that the reason was that Mormons do not smoke or drink. However, lots of people who get cancer do not smoke or drink, either. The difference is that the Mormon church preaches belonging to, and conducting oneself with consideration for, the group. Mormons are taught emotional entropy as part of their religion while the rest of us are all too often taught to feel like bigots if we believe our roots and affiliations are of primary importance.

As groups get blended into the melting pot, the individual's sense of dissociation can result in a greater incidence of distortion of emotional entropy and thus cancer. When Americans lived more in separate ethnic communities, the cancer rate was lower. At this time in our history, the extended family was also common. Mothers were not alone with their young. A sister-in-law lived upstairs. A grandmother or an aunt lived with the family or nearby. When the irritation of raising a newborn became overwhelming, someone stepped in to help. They did not ask permission; they simply took over for a while. The new mother's irritation was thus diminished, and she could more easily relate lovingly to her infant.

There are other categories of people who tend to be precancerous. There is a higher incidence of cancer among the young. In the case of youth, the rate of growth, while less rapid than in the newborn, is still high. But more important, any behaviorist will tell you that habit strength or learning is most intense the closer it is in time to the original conditioning. The fact that so many youngsters get pervasive cancer seems to indicate the power of autistic stage learning. Leukemia is all too common in young people. The white blood cells intended to protect us from invaders instead are reproduced cancerously.

The elderly have the highest incidence of cancer. It is safe to assume that translocations can more easily be activated with the vulnerability that age brings on. Even middle age provides evidence of this increasing vulnerability. In women over thirty-five, the chromosomes start to degenerate, leading to translocations of the genes in the ova and subsequent birth defects. The immune system becomes less efficient as people age, but, what is most important is the fact that the elderly have usually lost significant relationships through the deaths of loved ones. The survivors suffer the abrupt ending of emotional entropic systems. How many times have we heard of an elderly husband dying, followed almost immediately by the wife's developing cancer?

The sudden end of an entropic relationship seems to tip the scales. However, prolonged existence without such a fusion causes even individuals outside the usual categories to be vulnerable. Serial relationships and promiscuity indicate an inability to relate intimately. Sexual gratification is very different from the intense fusional love that sex can facilitate in an entropic relationship.

Reoccurrence of herpes is far more frequent in people with self-contained entropic defenses. The AIDS syndrome occurs primarily in sexually promiscuous homosexual males. The lack of an entropic relationship makes the individual more vulnerable.

Emotional entropy may be viewed as the central processor of all kinds of irritation. It bridges the gap between the biochemistry and psychology of human existence. The concept of emotional entropy integrates nutritional, viral, and genetic theories of the causes of cancer with circumstantial life events. The awareness of the existence of the precancerous personality permits us to take preventative measures against the disorder.

8

Prevention of Cancer During Rapid Growth Periods

TRYING TO AVOID EXTERNAL carcinogens is like an old deer trying to outrun a wolf pack. A burst of speed may help for a while, but then the pack encircles its victim and moves in. There is no escape.

It is clear that we cannot successfully avoid all contact with external irritants. This is not to say we should not work to minimize contact with them or to clean up the environment. But until our society is truly committed to cleaning up its technological act, attempting to avoid carcinogens is equivalent to whistling in a very polluted wind! Obviously no one should expose himself to these agents any more than necessary, but some exposure is unavoidable.

Obsession with the problem is in itself a stimulator of internal irritants. Worrying is a trait of the precancerous personality. It only serves to pollute an individual from the inside! At least if we can minimize the production of these internal pollutants, we will not be adding to the external ones.

There are four categories of life events that are significant in the evolution of cancer. They have similar biological and psychological processes taking place at the same time. Biologically, the cells are dividing rapidly and new cellular growth is taking place, not just replacement of worn-out cells. Elevated hormone levels apparently trigger the reaction.

Psychologically, what is particularly striking about these four categories is the preponderance of autistic residuals. In all four categories, the individuals involved share a lower level of emotional defenses, a tendency to be self-contained, a drifting in and out of contact with the world at large, a hypersensitivity to irritation, and the possibility of depression.

The four categories are:

1. Infancy
2. Pregnancy
3. Adolescence
4. Sickness or injury

In all of these categories, mitosis (cell division) is largely modulated by elevated hormone levels. In all of these categories, we are dealing with either the newborn psyche directly or its residuals. Emotionally, autistic functioning appears to be tied into this biological growth and/or healing process. All of these categories have an intrinsic potential for emotional and biological danger.

This union of emotional regression with rapid cell division we will call psychoplasia. It is not known which causes which, but they must occur together to facilitate efficient growth and healing. Psychoplasia is a universal human experience. We all go through it at various points in our lives.

Again, let us start at the beginning. The baby is the human being at the most sensitive and thus most vulnerable point in life. His sensory systems are more like those of lower animals at this stage than at any other. Sensitivity to chemical and physical irritants is extremely high. The baby is highly cooperative in letting us know when he has had too much stimulation. His discomfort at being overstimulated, either internally or externally, is obvious. The internal irritations of growth have a limited number of discharge mechanisms. He can use his voluntary muscles in apparently random movements for the purpose of dissipation, but the effective discharge through the fusional relationship of mother and baby is better still. All of this has been discussed previously. What still remains to be gone into are the means of lowering irritation for the newborn.

Most important, *no one should worry about spoiling a newborn baby.* This is a psychological absurdity. This tiny human has no concept of cause and effect. His connections with the world can be made only through the autonomic areas of the nervous system, and any learning or conditioning that takes place at this time will be within this system. This is the time when he needs the most protection from irritation.

The newborn should be fed on demand as his system requires. If not, the first psychological message that he receives in life is that he was born to meet the needs of others. This evolves into the basic anxiety so many of us suffer from. Anxiety in new parents can result in finding comfort in rigidity. But scheduled feedings for the newborn are an invitation for hyperirritation and translocations in the developing digestive tract and related systems.

The only mothers who can let their newborns continue to scream in pain are those whose pediatricians have told them, "This is what is best for the kid. Let him cry himself to sleep. If you let him do it a couple of times, he will stop carrying on."

I am sure the doctor is correct. The baby will eventually stop carrying on. But at what price? The price may be a dynamic for cancer.

Hospital procedures in this regard are highly questionable. In some instances, newborns are not fed for eight, ten, or even twelve hours while nurses wait for the first bowel movement to ascertain that the digestive tract is unblocked.

Any adult going that long without food would certainly protest. Just listen to yourself or friends who are dieting. For a baby, this is a horrendous amount of irritation immediately after birth.

Whenever I hear the term overstimulation being applied to the

113

newborn, I immediately think in terms of hyperirritation. Over-stimulation is overloading the capacity of the baby's nervous system by stimulation that seems at times unrelenting. Usually the overstimulation occurs because the baby's needs are subordinated to those of the parents. An extreme example is a young father insisting that it is all right to take his two-week-old daughter into a smoky poolroom bar. A more common example is awakening the baby to entertain the grandparents or other relatives.

Internal stimuli can be dealt with in overstimulating ways, also. If a parent goes overboard trying to soothe a crying baby, patting and jiggling and bouncing him around with no success, he may be surprised to find that when he gives up in despair and puts the baby down, the baby will go right to sleep.

The baby can recover from other errors but not from being left alone or being ignored during times of hyperirritation. Parents must be flexible in trying to find new ways to soothe the baby. If it is not food that he wants, perhaps he needs changing. Or the baby may be too hot or too cold. Or he may simply need to be held and cuddled. The baby may also respond to soothing words or a lullaby. Above all, the parent should respond to the baby in a relaxed and sympathetic way. A frantic reaction just adds irritation to the irritation the baby already is suffering from. Remember, crying is almost the only way the baby has of communicating.

Mistakes within reasonable limits in caring for the baby physically are of almost no significance if a fusion is taking place. If, however, there is minimal emotional entropy, then even minor physical errors in infant care may be experienced as gross irritations. The mother (or mother substitute) must be capable of loving the newborn or serious consequences ensue. Love is not optional in childrearing. It is vitally necessary for survival as was documented in a study done by René Spitz in 1947 (see chapter

12). The baby's resistance to accepting love after being taught to fear this closeness is very similar to the cancer patient's dynamic.

The second category is pregnancy, including the months immediately thereafter. For our purposes, we should think of pregnancy lasting at least a year. For the protection of the health of both the baby and the mother, it is essential to provide proper care and emotional feeding of the expectant and new mother to facilitate the emotional regression on her part necessary for fusion with the baby.

Pregnancy and the early mothering experience necessitates the shifting back and forth from autistic functioning (hypersensitivity, mood swings, dissociation, etc.) to more adult functioning. At the same time, the pregnant woman is undergoing rapid mitotic growth. Like the newborn, she experiences intense autistic feelings as she undergoes rapid cell division. She is undergoing psychoplasia, also.

It is unfortunately easy for a husband, friends, or relatives to dismiss or even become angry with the strange behavior of an adult expressing infantile feelings. But a husband should never say to his pregnant wife, "You're only feeling this way because you're pregnant." She does not care why she is feeling what she is feeling. She needs to have her feelings respected and soothed.

When autistic residuals are activated in the expectant or new mother, they limit the importance of words in the expression of caring. Close physical contact and gestures of unsolicited giving are far more soothing. How one says something, the tone, the feeling behind it, is far more important than the words themselves.

Women need to feel protected and cared for at this vulnerable time, but some have extremely powerful defenses against such feelings. They may find them too frightening and therefore deny them. They will even be offended by the idea that they should have such feelings.

As such a defensive new mother asserts her need for total self-control, one should avoid any confrontation. Instead, husband and family should be particularly considerate and complimentary while trying to persuade the mother to allow them to share in the care of the new baby.

When the new mother is experiencing infantile feelings, and perhaps acting on some of them, it is vitally important for the husband not to add to any upset. His task is to minimize irritation, not to make it worse. But merely not adding irritation to the hyperirritated state is not enough. The intensity must be lowered. The most effective way is through an entropic relationship. *The key to cancer prevention is the minimizing of any and all irritations at all stages of life.* This is best done through the processes of emotional entropy and fusion.

An area of special consideration is adoption. Adoptive mothers can regress to permit a fusion or they may resist. If the regression does take place, it is a sudden shock to the system. This new mother feels all the feelings of the biological mother but far more powerfully and abruptly. It is an overnight condensation of what should have taken nine months. Cancer is not related to adoption. It is related to the fusion or lack of it between *any* mother and her newborn baby.

Marilyn is a thirty-two-year-old who has adhesions in both fallopian tubes, probably, because of some earlier undetected infection. After surgical attempts to remove the adhesions, she was still infertile. She and her husband applied for adoption through a church facility. Three and a half years later, they were suddenly notified that a baby was available for them. Two days later, little Eric was brought home.

Marilyn reported what seemed like bizarre feelings, but they actually fit right into the concept of maternal regression to autism. She said, "I had almost four years to prepare for Eric's arrival. I wanted this baby more than anything in my life. John, my husband, had expressed similar feelings and was very sympa-

thetic to my need for a baby. Can you imagine his reaction when, on the way to the adoption agency, I told him that I just could not do it, that I was terrified and I did not know why. He parked the car and tried to reason with me. Then he just hugged me and said we could wait a day or so and make up our minds. I began to cry hysterically. I couldn't stop. I told him that I really felt totally wacko because now I could go through with it.

"When the nun handed me the baby, I had the strangest sensation that he was melting into me and vice versa. It was such a delicious sensation. He nestled right into my arms and chest. It was love at first sight. At home, I was a real character. I wouldn't let anyone feed the baby, not even John, for two days. He somehow seemed to understand. He stayed home from work and took care of me, instead. When I finally collapsed he was right there for both of us. I continued to have some really strange reactions.

"I developed a rash because of the soap I had been using. As soon as I switched to another brand, the rash went away. For several weeks after Eric's birth, I could not have sexual intercourse. It made me very uncomfortable, but I managed to satisfy John in other ways. What was strange was that I behaved like a seductive kitten, but I could not tolerate being penetrated. At times I cried for no reason. Everything seemed to upset me. I really thought I was losing it!"

Marilyn's reactions are understandable if we put them in the context of the primary maternal regression and fusion with her son Eric. Her husband, John, was intuitively excellent at meeting her primitive emotional needs. He did not once attack her throughout her adjustment to the regression. He somehow knew that what she was going through could not be dealt with through reasoning. Instead of being antagonistic, he supported her in whatever feelings she experienced.

John said that he was really frightened for her and that he felt totally inadequate and did not know what to do. He may not have *known* what to do, but he did have all the right feelings to help mother his wife at this critical time. Eric is now six years old. He is a delightful child, quite capable of having and appropriately expressing all of his feelings.

Adoption should occur as soon after birth as possible. Agencies that require a waiting period may be assisting in the development of, at the least, genetic translocations. The consequences may be far more severe. Any policy that interferes with the immediate fusion of a newborn and its mother, biological or adoptive, should be abolished.

Marilyn's reaction to Eric is, unfortunately, not the usual reaction of adoptive mothers. The adoption agency typically tells the adoptive mother that she and her husband have been selected because of their maturity. No one has told her that part of being mature is being accepting of all one's feelings, even the infantile emotions. If she begins to feel the discomfort of a sudden regression, she immediately turns it off. If she has other significant pressures, such as an immature, withholding husband or a need to return to work at the earliest possible date, she is in no position to accept a regression.

Child-custody cases can raise serious problems for babies and small children. The children should never suffer the abrupt termination of a fusion deliberately. Even in cases of abuse, the only reason to separate a mother and a small child is if the abuse is life threatening. What may appear to be a terrible relationship is in most instances better than the shock of an abrupt end to even such a limited emotional entropic system. The most important consideration in child abuse in general is that the mother's sense of isolation breeds abuse.

The next category that experiences intermittant emotional regression to autism coupled with increased hormone levels and rapid mitotic growth is adolescence. Adolescence is a period of psychoplasia in everyone's life. As an individual approaches and passes puberty, a significant increase in hormones of many kinds results in a general growth spurt and the development of secondary sexual characteristics. Overnight the eleven- or twelve-year-old may appear to change into a semiadult. Boys develop an increased muscle bulk, broadened shoulders, body hair, and enlargement of sexual organs. Girls develop their breasts and hips and begin their menstrual cycle.

Volumes have been written about the teenager, who is perhaps one of the least understood individuals in the world. Temper tantrums and depressions, infatuations and promiscuity, delinquency and righteousness are all part of the same beast. Teenagers can be space cadets. We talk to them and notice two minutes later that they have heard nothing we said. They can spend long hours in isolation pursuing hobbies, studying, or looking out the window. They switch dramatically from extroversion to introversion. They are moody; feelings are intense, extreme, and at times overwhelming.

Teenagers may do things that seem absurdly provocative and have no explanation whatsoever. Bodily sensations may seem overpowering. Hyperactivity is also characteristic of the adolescent, and they can eat enormous quantities of food without becoming obese. This unbounded energy and activity level is vitally important, for it allows the dissipation of autistic level irritations through the voluntary musculature. It may very well be life preserving.

Athletic pursuits are vital to teenagers, but walking into town with friends and hanging out is also. This need for activity is a lifesaving defense for the hyperirritated baby in a somewhat adult body.

Adolescents are often clumsy, and they go through periods of immature levels of motor coordination. Usually we blame this on rapid growth, but it is similar to the lack of coordination and clumsiness observed in schizophrenics. The teenager and the schizophrenic on the autistic level are both clumsy because their mental and biological regressions bring them at times to infantile levels of coordination.

119

The teenager's other major defense against the evolution of cancer is first love. A pressing need for emotional entropy is activated by the adolescent's psychobiological regression to autism. But parents are no longer suitable for such intense fusion. The more mature parts of both teenagers and parents cannot tolerate the overstimulation of two sexually adult people being so intimate when sex is a taboo. So first love steps in as a replacement for parental intimacy from the infantile stage of life.

The teenager needs this fusion in order to deal with his hyper-irritation, for the emotional pressures of adolescence create an overabundance of endogenous carcinogens.

If parents realize what is happening to the teenager, they do not have to feel injured by normal lack of connection or consideration of parents on the part of teenagers.

If there was not an adequate fusion in infancy, certain problems may develop in adolescence. Alcohol, marijuana, cocaine, barbiturates, etc., all assist in dulling the senses to overwhelming irritation from the inside or the outside. Unfortunately most teenagers do experiment with drugs, but continuous and excessive indulgence indicates a pressing need to turn off the hypersensitivity of autism.

The disturbed teenager can endure the endogenous carcinogen factory of a competitive and pressurized school situation if he has just smoked a joint. Without it, he will climb the walls.

Drugs appear, superficially, to be a facilitator of social interaction. In reality, the result is greater self-containment. Excessive drug use is a symptom of an inability to fuse, which may relate to subsequent cancer.

Sexual promiscuity, which is very common in adolescence, is another result of inadequate fusion in infancy.

Union with one individual is one mechanism for fusion. The teenager also has an avid need to belong in general. Special groups form to meet such needs. This even explains the importance of athletic teams, sororities and fraternities, and high school and college clubs. As with the Mormons, belonging is the dominant theme. If a teenager does not or cannot experience first love or intense, at times seemingly fanatic, group membership, it may indicate an inability to fuse and, thus, an aberrant emotional entropic system.

Inability to relate on such a level frequently results in moderate to dangerously severe depressions. These depressions are an attempt to ward off hyperirritation. Increased hormone levels are irritants or internal carcinogens. An anaclitic depression (see chapter 12) serves to minimize outside emotional irritants to avoid a repetition of the hyperirritability of early infancy, but at the same time, it maximizes endogenous carcinogens.

Like the anaclitically depressed baby or cancer patient, the adolescent will push the concerned individual away. Concern is viewed as intrusive. How many times have parents heard, "You just don't understand me. I can't talk to you." This translates to: You don't love me, and I cannot tolerate your intrusions!

This pushing away can eventually lead to totally self-contained hyperirritation, which can be fatal. In adolescence it leads to suicide, which can be either conscious and direct (pills, guns, hanging, etc.) or unconscious and indirect (auto accidents, overdoses, provoked homicide, leukemia, etc.).

As the adolescent's cells reproduce, there is a risk of additional translocations in the organ systems forming new tissue. This is true of any neoplasia. But unlike the newborn, adolescents, pregnant women, and the sick or injured do have psychological defenses that, at least, are thought to help process irritation. The more mature individual can escape or defend against these powerful irritations; so it is not new translocations that are the predominant issue here. It is the hyperirritability that stems from the increase in hormone levels and the discomforts of rapid mitotic growth ("growing pains"). The psychoplasia of more advanced life stages is not nearly as severe as in the first two months of life, but it does make an individual more vulnerable to the elevated irritation levels tripping a land mine laid in infancy.

Thus the adolescent needs to be protected from the physical damage to which the anaclitic depression is related. The wise parent or teacher at this time will not add irritation to preexisting irritation. He will not put the baby down, even though the baby is now thirteen, sixteen, or eighteen years of age.

However, this time around, it is even more difficult. This baby can be devastating in his ability to push away obnoxiously. He can get his parents and teachers to want, not only to go along with putting him down, but he can get them actually to want to kill him at times!

If the anaclitic depression cannot be resolved by the parents (if they cannot make contact with the teenager), then professional help is a necessity. Permitting long term isolation is a repetition of the infantile dynamic of self-containment. It can be fatal.

Less severe but very significant is the basic parent-teenager conflict. Anytime you attempt to coerce an adolescent, you are probably adding to irritation. This is not to suggest that limits should not be set to adolescent behavior. They indicate a love and concern that adolescents can sense. If, however, they are set as part of a power play, they become unbearable irritants that result in rebellion. Teenagers cannot be told to do something without an adequate explanation without having them develop powerful resentments. It is far better to work toward cooperation.

The following is an example of how not to add irritation to preexisting adolescent irritation.

Robert is a thirty-eight-year-old dentist with a private practice and an office in his home. His daughter Judy is a fifteen-year-old high school student. On Wednesdays and Fridays, Robert gives her a ride home from school since he has ten minutes free between patients. Judy is usually five minutes late, which throws her father's schedule slightly off. In the past, he always attacked her for her apparently nonchalant attitude toward being late. She appeared to ignore him, which only made him angrier. On Wednesdays and Fridays, Judy became an unruly monster at home, picking on her little brother and/or retreating to her room.

Patient: Last Friday I tried what you suggested with Judy. Instead of attacking her right off for being late, I asked about it. She told me her last period teacher always keeps the class late. So I asked her if she ever explained the problem of my schedule. She told me she did, but her teacher did not seem to care. I then told her that this must create a lot of anxiety for her, being caught in the middle. She said it did. She told me at times she was nauseated by her Wednesday and Friday afternoons.

Analyst: Did you join her?

Patient: Did I ever! I told her that her teacher was being terrible to her and to me. I said I would write a note or speak to the principal. Then I added that the rotten so-and-so should be kicked out of the profession. I explained that by now this teacher knew the predicament she was in. I told her that it must be awful being made to sit for the five minutes and know she would be late. She told me it actually made her sick. I told her that I would talk to the school administration if need be. The amazing thing is what happened next. For the entire trip home Judy let loose with a stream of invective about this teacher and some of the others. The more she complained about them the happier she got. By the time we got home it was not my Wednesday-Friday Judy. She actually played with her brother and then offered to help him with his homework. Her stomachache disappeared in the car. She's been talking to me this week more than in the past year. She actually asked my opinion about some things. I couldn't believe my ears.

Analyst: What would have happened if you had continued with the usual position of attacking her for lateness?

Patient: She would have been bitchy all night and feeling sick. When I think of all the aggravation I caused her! I mean this teacher was busting her chops enough without me adding to it. It was miraculous what happened as soon as I did not add to it. I learned a lesson. I should say she taught me a lesson. Just think what she has been internalizing every Wednesday and Friday since September! Thanks for the advice. And I'm sure Judy's insides thank you, too.

What Robert did not realize was how profoundly inside his daughter's physiology the internalization took place. The genetic material of the nuclei of her cells was the possible degree of "insideness."

The final category of high risk for tripping a genetic land mine is convalescence. During convalescence the body is repairing itself (growing) through rapid cell division, which is largely under the influence of irritating natural chemical agents. At the same time, the activation of autistic residuals is taking place emotionally. An anaclitic depression may appear to be a defense against the overwhelming intensity of autistic feelings. The patient may, at times, push caring people away. He may be in and out of a comalike sleep. He may appear totally self-involved. He knows he should be interested in the life events of the friends and family who come to visit, but we can all recall visiting hospitals to see people we care about and suffering the discomfort of their forced involvement with our daily affairs, which seem mundane in the face of a coronary occlusion, for instance.

Even with less severe injury or illness, most of us regress to self-involvement. The definitive indicator of the regression to autism induced by physical trauma is the emotional symptom of being dissociated. The sick or injured are, at times, thoroughly

124

spaced out. Medication cannot account for all of these reactions; psychoplasia can.

One frequently hears it said in the waiting rooms of intensive care units, "Don't say anything to upset him!" In other words, do not add irritation to preexisting irritation.

When we visit a sick or injured person, we are naturally more tolerant of inappropriate comments coming from him. We put up with feeling rejected and pushed away by rationalizing that "Old Jim is just not himself." It is Old Jim, but it is also very *Young* Jim with whom we are dealing. This is why he seems unfamiliar.

Emotional entropy will assist healing as it assists growth. Healing can be viewed as new growth. Therefore, self-containment is to be avoided except for the periods of infantlike need for rest that accompany healing.

In most cases of healing and illness, the difficulty is in getting past infantile depression. We must be prepared to soothe the baby within the adult while these powerful feelings are laid bare.

9

Prevention of Cancer in Everyday Life

THIS CHAPTER IS ESPECIALLY for those of you who may have been reading this book and saying, "But I did many of those awful things to my babies." Don't worry. You can make amends.

The last chapter and this one will help you to recognize that internal levels of carcinogens in your loved ones and yourself are, to a great extent, under your control. The mechanisms of processing irritation can be relearned more easily in the young, but even the old can learn new tricks.

This chapter is about those new tricks.

Prevention in Childhood

The most carcinogenic statement that can be made to a child is, "Keep crying, and I'll give you something to cry about." This is the epitome of adding irritation to an already irritated human being. If you have been in the habit of saying things like this to your children, break the habit.

Normally, the degree of a parent's anger with a child will relate to the seriousness of the child's transgression, but nothing deserves this degree of upset. The child is already sufficiently disturbed. What he needs is comforting and soothing; the child does not need to be placed in an acutely hyperirritated state. If the child cannot expect love and soothing from his parents at these times, whom can he expect it from.

In a supermarket, a child's temper tantrum may seem like a public indictment to a parent—it can be very embarrassing. It is even more embarrassing if the tantrum has been caused by something the parent has said or done. How should such situations be handled?

The most commonly accepted advice is to walk away and leave the child alone. Eventually, he will calm down. That is probably true. Just as the newborn will eventually cry himself to sleep if no one picks him up. Ignoring the toddler with a tantrum is just as harmful.

So, pick up the kicking, screaming toddler (he's a lot smaller than you are), hold him firmly, and speak to him soothingly, and eventually the screaming will turn to crying, the crying will turn to soft moaning, and the end result will be a peaceful child. There is no way to keep a child from ever being upset. Upsets will inevitably occur, and the only cure is love.

Parent's threats can certainly cause the overt symptoms of an upset to be buried—just think how far! It is this kind of induced hyperirritation that must be avoided. The parent's rage must be controlled or the child will have internal scars from it for life.

Have you ever said to your child, "Keep crying, and you will have to go to your room until you settle down?" This is not hyperirritation, it is true, but it is teaching self-containment. Most of us are guilty of this carcinogenic communication. It is the equivalent of leaving the baby to cry himself to sleep. The child needs his parents even if his crying is upsetting them. A temporarily irritated parent is better than an emotionally exiled child.

However, while separation is undesirable because it means self-containment and isolation for the child, it is perhaps better than the cumulative addition of irritation that would occur if the parent heaps his or her upsets on the already irritated child.

Consider another situation. Imagine being a three-year-old who is afraid of the dark because of the lurking monsters, witches, and goblins. Where are yours? Perhaps in the closet, so that those doors have to be shut each night. Maybe they hide under your bed or are just outside the window.

Shadows conceal evil somethings for most of us. When you admitted your fears to your mother and father, the conversation may have gone something like this:

Child: Daddy, I'm scared of the dark. I don't want you to go. Please don't.

Father: What are you afraid of in the dark?

Child: There's a green thing that is over there (pointing to the closet). I'm scared of it. It's ugly.

Father: (Laughing) There are no such things. That's all make-believe. There's nothing to be afraid of. Now, you just get into bed and go to sleep. I'll be downstairs so don't worry.

Child: Please, Daddy, don't go!

Father: It's all make-believe. Now, you stop it and go to sleep. I'll leave the hallway light on. *Don't be scared.*

What this father did not take into account is the importance of magic in the development of all children. Magical thinking is a major part of the preschooler's existence. When you ignore it for fear of encouraging it, you are inadvertently giving a communication that could be in a way carcinogenic.

When the father walked away from his child, he left the youngster in a state of terror. He also left the child alone in a hyperirritated state, thus, reinforcing self-containment.

How could this be handled better?

Child: Daddy, I'm scared of the dark! I don't want you to go. Please don't!

Father: What are you afraid of in the dark? When I was your age I was afraid of monsters and witches in the dark. Mine were blue with red eyes and red teeth. What are yours like?

Child: Mine are green with big hands. They come out of my closet at night. I'm scared of them, Daddy!

Father: Let me teach you some secret words. Whenever you see a monster, say these words and the monster will turn into a nice fairy. The words are boo, boo, who. Say them back to me.

Child: Boo, boo, who. Boo, boo, who. Boo, boo, who.

Father: Now, remember them. The monsters change right away. Now, I'll check the closet before I leave. Remember, the magic words are boo, boo, who. If you need me, call. I'll be right here. But I know that boo, boo, who always work.

Child: Daddy, please tuck me in.

A couple reported to me that their two-year-old was frightened by the imaginary spiders in her room, and every night there was a battle to get the child to go to bed. I suggested the use of the Tasmanian devil, a character from the Bugs Bunny cartoons who viciously devours anything in sight that has carbon atoms in it. They bought a stuffed animal version of the devil and told their daughter that this evil-looking creature would take care of her. While she slept, the Tasmanian devil would eat all the spiders in her room.

The couple reported that they had total success with the devil, with one interesting side effect. Little Samantha is an angelic-looking blond-haired, green-eyed child. She has grown so attached to "Tassie," as she calls her protector, that this ugly monster has replaced her teddy bear. She takes the creature everywhere with her and gets tremendous attention from people, who are unable to reconcile the contrast between the beautiful Samantha and her Tassie.

Using magic in the face of magical thinking reduces hyperirritated states. It provides protection by the parent in the form of magical phrases or protective stuffed animals. Most parents are afraid that this will convince their children that magic is true. That won't happen. To children at certain stages, magic is the only truth in the face of fear of annihilation. However, children outgrow it. But in a stressful situation, we may all regress to it, later in life.

For example, imagine yourself in the Battle of the Bulge with a panzer tank coming right at you. If you are like many people, you might very well call for your mother in the face of such terror. The magical part would be ascribing omnipotence to her. After all, how good is she with a bazooka or grenades? During such regressive fear, the need is to seek a magical savior. The farther back the regression, the more likely that mother will be called for.

The child encounters his panzer tank every night. Don't desert him when he faces such terror. He will abandon the need for a magical savior with age. That is not the issue. What is important is what you are teaching him throughout this stage: the choice between self-containment, which can be carcinogenic, and fusion, which is not.

In introducing a child to any recreational activity that you enjoy, there is a secret to success that prevents both of you from becoming hyperirritated. The first time, the parent is not there to enjoy it. The parent's sole function, if he or she wants the child to become an eventual companion in this activity, is to be there to comfort and encourage the child. If the parent is deluded into thinking that he or she is there to enjoy the activity, also, conflicts will arise.

A man told me how he, at first, turned off his daughter to the fishing he so much enjoyed but, eventually, wound up with a fishing buddy. On the first visit to the lake, he quickly showed the girl where the bass would most likely be, the proper way to cast, and what bait to use. He was in a hurry to get this over with so that he could go after the monster fish that stole his favorite lure the previous week. After about ten minutes of fishing, he saw his daughter sitting down moping. He told her to keep trying, that it takes patience. She refused. He got angry, and the day ended with neither of them speaking to the other.

The next time out, he put the tackle on the ground, and they sat on the shore. He began skipping pebbles on the lake, and his daughter joined in the game. When she got bored, they hiked around the lake. He never mentioned fishing, but to his amazement, she asked to try the pretty lure with all the bright colors. He knew it was the wrong choice but tied it on for her anyway. When she made her first catch, both she and the fish were hooked. Best of all, only the fish was hyperirritated.

To teach a new behavior pattern requires many repetitions of stimulus-response groups. You cannot expect a child to learn anything based upon one or two episodes. If you are guilty of isolated incidents of encouraging your child to learn self-containment, remember that it is Hollywood that makes singular traumas the significant part of learning. In reality, you must repeat and repeat. If your baby was conditioned into fusion, occasional mistakes will be of little consequence.

What if you recognize now that your child was conditioned into self-containment in the face of hyperirritation? Reconditioning can provide a possible way out. If you stop reinforcing the self-containment, you will gradually take away the motivation, and the child's behavior can change.

Mary's usual behavior was to withdraw to her room whenever her father tried to offer constructive criticism of her behavior. Her father was afraid that if he tried to persuade her to stay with him to talk the matter over she would begin not to take his criticism seriously. But rather than worry about sending mixed messages to his daughter, he should have encouraged her to remain with him to communicate about the feelings they were each experiencing.

If a parent's interactions with his child have been predominantly carcinogenic, all it takes is occasional intermittant rein-forcement to keep it carcinogenic. So it is important to work to avoid these episodes. The parent must learn to respond to hyper-irritation without adding to it and to self-containment in such a way as to encourage communication. The child must not be allowed to retreat into himself.

Consider this common situation. The playroom is always a mess. Charles habitually leaves all of his toys on the floor, some-times in dangerous locations. His parents have tried punishment and threats to get him to pick up and put his toys where they belong. Typically Charles refuses to cooperate or does it so slowly that his mother is reduced to vindictive attacks on her ten-year-old.

A better way to handle this situation would go something like this:

Mother: It isn't going to work anymore.
Charles: What isn't going to work anymore?
Mother: You think that if you leave these toys around I am going to keep screaming at you about it. Well, I am not. I want you to tell me why you want me to scream at you.
Charles: I never want you to scream at me.
Mother: If you don't want me to scream at you, it takes about three to five minutes to pick up all your toys. It is just not going to work anymore. There will be no screaming over this sort of situation. If you cooperate with me, I will cooperate with you. You want to go to the movies this weekend. I am certain I will be more likely to do what you want if you can do a little bit of what I want. If not, that is okay. We don't have to go to the movies.

No matter what, the mother is not going to allow herself to lose her temper. She is now aware that, for some reason, this is what Charles wants of her, and she is going to ruin his game.

133

Help remove some hyperirritated states, and your child will seek you out. This is reconditioning. Many positive repetitions are necessary to effect relearning. On the other hand, few are necessary to reinforce what already has been negatively learned. It all boils down to stopping the negative episodes and beginning a positive reeducation at the same time.

I was sitting in a family restaurant on Long Island, and a rather nice-looking, affluent young family was at the next table. Their adorable child was busy being a four-year-old.

Four is a transitional age, something like eleven or twelve. These are ages between important stages. They bridge the gaps in childhood development. For this reason, they can be difficult times for the child and the parents. The striving for maturity and independence is coupled with earlier, less mature patterns. There is confusion on everyone's part. Experts and laymen alike tend to see these stages as developmental no-man's-lands.

This particular four-year-old was busily playing with his food and having a wonderful time. His mother kept telling him to stop playing and sit quietly. She warned him that if he kept fooling around with food in his mouth he would choke. It was almost as if she had ordained it.

The next instant he was trying to clear his throat of the food he was choking on. The father, who, I later found out, was a physician, smacked the little boy's back, and the food came up. The mother reacted in what seemed like an inexcusable way: as the child was crying, frightened, and gasping for air, she screamed and shook him violently.

This is the epitome of adding irritation to irritation. It is also conditioning the child to not show feelings nor to expect or want comfort when hyperirritated.

However, one swallow does not a summer make. If the mother normally reacted this way, this child would certainly be damaged. But if we take into consideration how terrified *she* was, we can understand and forgive the isolated transgression. She should also forgive herself.

On the other hand, if this child's autistic-stage conditioning was precancerous, then intermittent episodes like this would reinforce the conditioning. For the mother to counteract the earlier conditioning, she must learn to offer comfort in the face of hyperirritation.

After the child settles down, is gently hugged and stroked, she can tell him: "I was frightened when you choked. Please don't play with food like that anymore. This is what can happen. I bet it scared you, too!" The child would probably react by talking about how frightened he was while describing his hyperirritated state. The internal irritants would immediately subside as his mother caresses him and wipes away his tears. She will have dissipated their effect.

Perhaps the more subtle continuation of negative early stage learning occurs in hostile or negligent marital situations. Either parent can be guilty. If your marriage is hard to tolerate at times, ask yourself if you have been using your children to meet the emotional needs your spouse should be meeting. If a spouse is absent because of death or divorce, the risk of doing this is even greater.

In this situation, the child may be pushed into the position of assuming the adult emotional role in place of the absent parent. The child not only learns to delight in taking care of the parent's needs but also gets rewarded for it. The child begins to feel responsible for any upsets the parent experiences. The child sits and listens to mother's or father's complaints and almost never gets to express his or her own. When the parent becomes depressed, the child may not feel responsible for the cause but can feel guilt over not being able to remove the depression.

In this kind of situation, parents will express pride in the fact that their child is ten years old going on thirty—a most depressing thing to hear anyone say about any child. It indicates the possibility that not only is the child being conditioned for self-containment but is also being denied childhood. Anyone brought up this way will have the idea that being mature means denying all infantile or childish feelings, while genuine maturity is based upon being able to acknowledge all of your thoughts and feelings but acting upon them selectively. The child of a parent who becomes emotionally dependent on him fears that childlike behavior will result in estrangement from the parent who needs his care.

Usually the child cares for only one parent, and he identifies with this parent's resentment of the other one. The rejected parent may then resort to distancing himself or herself from the child. A father may see the child as belonging to the mother and have nothing more to do with the child.

The situation can become very difficult to correct, but both parents should make every attempt to do so, however great the emotional strain. The parent who is reversing roles with the child must find a new emotional support system. The distancing parent must draw closer and let the child know that he or she is always there.

Not every bad marriage or divorce evolves into a subtly destructive situation that refreshens precancerous conditioning. But it is something to be seriously considered by anyone in this unhappy life circumstance.

On the other hand, do not overcompensate by never allowing your children to do anything for you. It is the direction of the emotional entropy that counts. Children need the parent to absorb their irritation, not vice versa. Immature parents are always a problem for the development of healthy children. Occasional immature behavior (inappropriate venting of rage, asking a child's opinion about matters he should not have to be concerned with, etc.) are insignificant if the autistic-stage conditioning had the emotional entropic system going in the right direction. But the child who has always had to worry about a parent's reaction will, in later life, generally be hyperirritated internally by worrying about everyone's potential reactions. As an adult, he will be overly concerned about doing the right thing and making the right impression. What an enormous strain this is on anyone unfortunate enough to have been so conditioned.

In discussing childrearing, the matter of corporal punishment cannot be avoided. Is it ever appropriate to strike a child? Many say absolutely not. Others say that it is sometimes the only way to get your message across. Both positions are wrong. Hitting a child should be reserved only for one of two reasons.

1. To be protective in life threatening situations—A two-year-old does not have the thought development to know that his mother does not want him in the street because a truck could run over him without the driver even knowing it. He cannot understand that apartment windowsills are not for climbing on. He cannot know that abusing the family Doberman can get him killed. He *can* know that Mommy will smack his rear if he does any of those things. Inflict just enough pain to cause discomfort and fear of your reaction to any of the child's life-threatening pursuits. In these situations the child should fear the parent. He cannot fear the real dangers until it is too late.

It is true to some degree that hitting the child will result in possible hyperirritation. But if your two-year-old does wind up under the truck or car or face down in the swimming pool, we do not have to worry about subsequent cancer, do we? In addition, the child who is transgressing in life-endangering ways is not usually in a preexisting state of hyperirritation. The added irritation is sudden and pronounced, but it is not added to a hyperirritated mind or body. The child will understand that he is being protected and not punished.

A caution: Many people believe that allowing a child to touch a hot stove or radiator, even if it results in blistered skin, will teach a beneficial lifetime lesson. In addition to the excruciating pain inflicted on the child, it also carries the terrible message that mother, who is responsible for his protection, let this happen. A child must never deliberately be allowed to hurt himself.

2. If you tend to lose control and be physically and emotionally abusive—In this situation, the intent is to avoid resorting to significant emotional and physical abuse. If you know that you can lose control and that you usually do, consider this: Before you are so out of control that abuse will follow, give the child a less severe smack on the backside. This can help put the brakes on for both of you. Telling anyone who is overly severe with a child just to stop is a waste of time. Venting some rage, but in a controlled way, is far more likely to work. Everyone wants to abuse their children at times, and almost everyone does to some degree.

Hitting can thus be viewed as a medicine, and all medicines have some potentially negative side effects. It is important to weigh the risks versus the benefits much like a physician must do in treating any disease or disorder.

The two most important points to remember in raising children are:

1. Avoid adding irritation to preexisting irritation.
2. Avoid self-containment of irritation.

If you follow these rules, you are very likely avoiding interactions related to cancer. And you are most certainly providing the child with an orientation in life that will assist him or her in maturing and relating to others in a constructive manner.

Do not expect to be able to do a perfect job. But the more you try, the more benefits you will see.

Prevention during Marriage
If there is one basic tenet to follow for a marriage to be an efficient emotional entropic system it is this: *Feelings take precedence over facts.*

In troubled marriages, someone is always wrong and someone

is always right. The need to prove this indicates an investment in power plays and dominance. *There is no right or wrong in a marriage.* The only significant aspect of conflict is the feeling surrounding it. If feelings are dealt with first, the facts are almost always more easily resolved. If, however, one partner *needs* to be right all the time, the relationship can easily become disastrous. When one spouse denigrates or ignores the other's feelings, the conditioning for self-containment is activated. A husband may dismiss his wife's hurt feelings as ridiculous and not worth discussing. A wife may ignore a husband's needs as unimportant. Whatever the mechanism for wiping out feelings in a relationship, a relationship without feelings is wiped out!

You may consider your partner's position on an issue absurd. In reality it may be absurd. But reality quite possibly has nothing to do with the feelings involved. If you resort to *inflicting* your reality upon the situation, you are encouraging hyperirritation and self-containment in the other.

If your partner has to be overly concerned about your reactions to different issues, then the emotional entropy is going in one direction. The partner who is more mature and in better control of himself or herself will be the one more likely to get cancer.

The marital relationship should ideally permit comfortable expression of feelings and thoughts from both partners. If a great disparity of maturity exists, then the more mature partner will be continually looking out for the other's feelings. The fragility and vulnerability of the immature partner will necessitate such care. This repeats the early infantile-maternal relationship. If this repetition occurs for only one partner, the other will have no means within the relationship of having his or her emotional irritation dealt with. He or she will remain self-contained as it becomes obvious over a period of time that the immature partner cannot deal with these feelings.

Precancerous individuals are excellent at caring for others but cannot accept unconditional caring directed toward them. Such a marriage may be comfortable. The partners may even have selected each other to fulfill these unconscious needs.

Sandra is fifty-two years old. She is a very proper woman who compulsively does everything right. Her husband, Ned, is a fifty-four-year-old stockbroker. His business is successful in spite of his obvious immaturity. At work he traffics in sexual byplay with his female staff. One secretary resigned because of his obnoxious behavior.

Whenever Sandra and Ned are out with friends, he is humorously seductive to any and all females, with the *exception* of his wife (mother). Sandra has repeatedly asked him to stop behaving this way, but he dismisses her feelings, saying, "You're so up tight! Can't you see I'm only kidding? I like to be lighthearted and have fun. You're such a stick in the mud."

Although his wife has pointed this out on many occasions, Ned refused to see that his behavior is felt by her as a hostile rejection. He insists that her perceptions are ridiculous. She can feel her insides knot up as she is coerced into ending the discussion.

Ned is an avid sports fan but prefers to worship his athletic heroes in the presence of men. Sandra has tried to be included. She knows major league statistics better than most men, and she can name players in the NFL based on numbers. But Ned claims that his friends tease him about his wife's attendance at games by asking if he always had his *mother* along.

Money is a constant source of conflict. Although Sandra pays all the bills, she has learned to get Ned's permission before buying anything for herself. If she does not, he flies into a rage.

It is easy to see that Sandra is at risk. Ned continually denigrates her, but he denies it if she points it out to him. He refuses to discuss any matter that is important to his wife. On the other hand, she never refuses his need to communicate. In fact she welcomes having any time to talk.

This marriage is carcinogenic because the emotional entropy is such that the irritation flows constantly from the husband to the wife. She absorbs it and contains it all within herself. Sandra would not dream of discussing her marital difficulties with anyone. On the surface her excuse is embarrassment. Beneath the surface is the fear of intimacy she suffers from. A marriage like this fits in perfectly with her autistic-stage conditioning. All irritation flows from him to her, and she must contain it or risk his elevated level of irritation being added to the irritation she already feels. Ned is her early mother. He will live to a ripe old age, while Sandra will probably succumb to cancer years earlier.

Whatever the problems are, no matter how absurd they appear to be, it is very important that a spouse always consider his or her mate's upset as the first order of business. The nature of the problem does not matter in the long run. It is how the two of them *process* marital irritation that does matter.

The following is another example of a couple in trouble:

Steven says that his wife, Helen, is totally lacking in passion. He feels unwanted because she shows no enthusiasm. He reports that she seems only to tolerate sexual contact. "She's so immature about it," Steven says, "that I feel like I am molesting a child." When he attempts to discuss this with Helen, it always turns out to be a monologue. She has nothing to say and remains unresponsive to any such discussions. If she does say anything at all, it is merely to say that she doesn't know why she can't respond. She feels attacked and belittled. Steven feels rejected and undesirable, but for the most part he tolerates and absorbs the irritation caused by her seeming lack of interest in a sexual relationship with her husband.

Helen never expresses closeness through sexual overtures. She cooks his favorite meals and tells him that that is proof that she cares for him. At such moments, Steven feels like choking on the food.

Steven is the far greater cancer risk of the two. He admits that many of the women he dated prior to Helen were sexually terrific. He then adds, appearing totally perplexed, that the more they made it clear that they genuinely cared about him and the more they took the sexual initiative to express love and devotion, the more he had a need to run. He even felt anger and disgust (a cover feeling for fear) at their expressions of love. Helen never behaved like this.

When they lie in bed at night, with Steven carrying on a monologue in his head about his problems and what he can do about them, he is once again a deserted, hyperirritated baby. He probably feels this way at the same time of night that he used to be left to cry himself to sleep.

Marriage can help reduce or add to our internal irritations, but marriage requires work to be anticancerous. Anticancerous marriage depends upon relative mutuality. If one spouse is the chronic giver and the other the receiver, a negative entropic system exists. Whether this centers on sex, the expression of feelings, or anything else, the system is one directional. After a time, the receiver may learn to resent the giver's inability to receive. It comes across as a lack of desire for whatever this person has to offer. More important, it induces guilt, which turns into a feeling of resentment, and then both partners become self-contained.

Patient: I'm married to the original Earth Mother. She does everything, and she does it right. I've never known anyone so giving and caring. The trouble is that she's zero at receiving. I mean she does not know how to make me feel appreciated or wanted.

Analyst: Most men would be content to have all their needs met.

Patient: You don't understand. She is great at meeting all my needs *but one.* I have a need to be appreciated and accepted for what I can do, for what I can express! You know something? In a sense, she's very selfish. She deprives me of one of the most important aspects of my life, and *I* feel guilty about it. I know she had a rough time growing up. She was always performing; the top of her class in high school. She keeps on performing and no one can get into her act. When I do something for her or give her a gift, I get the feeling that she is already trying to figure out how to outdo me! She cannot receive, and it is driving me crazy!

Anyone looking at this man's marriage superficially would assume that the wife is the giving, more mature partner. In reality she is a "performance-anxiety" baby. The husband's constant acceptance, with no mutuality, is necessary for her to feel valued. She thinks of herself as a very giving person. Little does she know that she is overwhelmingly demanding. The husband is at risk in this marriage.

The first step toward achieving an anticancer marriage rests upon communication, but unfortunately words are not enough. When it comes to avoiding cancer, feelings and actions can be even more important. Cancer stems from that time in life when we could not talk or understand language. All we could do was tune in to the feelings behind the words. In marriage words can be cheap. If the feelings and behavior do not change, all the talking in the world doesn't do any good.

Anticancer marriages are based upon feeling, behavior, and words. If a picture is worth a thousand words, a giving gesture in marriage is beyond value. When things are mutual and partners are equally mature, a great deal can be accomplished to assist each other in processing irritation through sharing. Sharing minimizes irritation; self-containment maximizes it.

If you do not have an anticancer marriage, work at it. If your spouse is uncooperative, you don't have to play the game by his or her rules. Your responses can help deal with the lack of cooperation. To begin with, do the opposite of what is expected. When he wants you distant and rejecting, be loving. Expect him to try to push you away. Don't fall for it! A reconditioning can happen if you don't respond as predicted. Throw the occasional curve ball. It can work wonders. Consider Paula and John:

John is the type of man who, when upset about business or any other significant matter in his life, retreats into himself. For years Paula interpreted this to mean that he didn't want to communicate with her, and she felt unwanted and rejected. She decided that something had to be done.

Rather than try to discuss the matter with him, something she had frequently tried before unsuccessfully, she managed to get past the symptoms and make physical contact with him when he was in his withdrawn moods. After several such significant preverbal and nonverbal interchanges, John almost miraculously began to talk about the problems that had caused his previous withdrawal and distancing.

The ideal anticancer marriage would have the following elements:

1. A shifting back and forth of the parental caring role.

2. Only one member of the couple would be angry at a time.

3. A desire to deal with and respect feelings as having priority over facts.

Shifting of parental roles in a marital relationship means that at different times irritation will be absorbed in different directions. Both will genuinely want to soothe each other with whatever works: talk, a hug, a giving gesture. Most important, both members of this team will provide this intimate caring when the other is hyperirritated. They will not permit retreat into self-containment.

Ideally only one partner in a marriage should get angry at a time so that the other can deal with the upset. If both are bordering on loss of control, then two hyperirritated babies are adding irritation to each other.

If facts predominate over feelings, then at least one partner will be more correct all the way to the divorce court. When you can stop and say that nothing is worth this pain and conflict, you are on your way to an anticancer marriage. When each of you, at different times and together, can put the brakes on and ask, "What are we really fighting over? What is worth such an upset?" you are in a very positive relationship.

All three of these elements are related to the basic anticancer premise of not adding irritation to irritation and at the same time combating self-containment. All three necessitate emotional entropy and fusion.

But even if a marriage fails to meet these needs, it apparently is better in many cases than having nothing. Remember that divorced and widowed women have a significantly higher incidence of breast and cervical cancer.

If remarriage occurs and is successful, a carcinogenic situation may have been avoided. The success of the remarriage may indicate that the need for a fusional relationship has finally been met. However, serial marriages suggest a strong possibility that an individual is unconsciously seeking fusionless relationships. It is a means of deceiving oneself. It is important to remember that we do what is familiar, not necessarily what is best for us. If this is your story, stop trying to fool yourself and recognize that you are avoiding intimacy.

Obviously not everyone in a carcinogenic relationship will get or induce cancer. It is all part of a constellation of dynamics that originates in infancy.

If your spouse develops cancer, it does not mean that you are the ogre who induced it. You are not responsible for establishing the autistic-stage translocations. You did not teach your spouse how to maximize irritants.

But guilt is always present when a loved one is seriously ill, injured, or dies. No two people can live together without having some hostile thoughts for the other one. Just don't give yourself so much credit or power as to assume you could induce cancer in anyone who was not set up for it years ago.

On a more superficial level, guilt or the reasons for it obviously are destructive to any marriage.

Prevention in Other Sexuality
Anything that is sexually pleasurable and agreeable to both parties, without causing pain, is potentially anticancer. However, recreational sex is just that: a recreation. It has little or nothing to do with emotional fusion, which only loving sexuality can promote. Orgasms can result in brief but powerful regression to the intense, unfocused state comparable to that of the autistic stage child. They can facilitate fusion or fight against it. They can become an object unto themselves, an end rather than a continuing means, with potentially disastrous effects.

Patient: I don't know what to do anymore. Most guys would be ecstatic to be in my shoes. Almost every night, I can go to bed with a different woman. Three cheers for the sexual revolution. The trouble is that I'm damned if I do and damned if I don't.

Analyst: Explain.

Patient: Well, before I make it with a woman, there is an excitement, the thrill of the hunt. I don't know. But if she tries to touch me after we have sex, my skin bristles! If she lights up a cigarette, I choke. I feel disgust at the touch

146

and smells of her body. I never feel this way before or during, just after. But the worst is that while she's telling me I was the greatest, I'm feeling really depressed. I mean *depressed*—Empty, hollow, like my insides fell out. The feeling is so unbearable that I commit the ultimate sin of the singles' world over and over: I screw and run. Sex for me is like fast food for most people. It is valueless nutritionally, it just fills you up. After a few weeks of heavy contact, I can't stand the depression anymore. I stop looking for new conquests. It hurts too much. I can't remember the last time I stayed overnight with anyone. I am never going to meet someone I can marry, not like this. I'll probably die young, single, alone.

This man is exhibiting the typical anaclitic depressive reaction as it pertains to sex. Sexual intimacy for him is superficial. He is thoroughly, though unconsciously, afraid of a genuine emotional attachment, but he realizes that his reactions are somehow wrong.

What we think of as old-fashioned romance may have developed out of human infantile conditioning for fusion. Romance may be viewed as a repetition of the mother and child falling in love and getting used to each other. In the adolescent and adult version, the mother and newborn roles switch back and forth between the partners. When people get to know each other before they go to bed together, they have a much better chance of developing emotional entropy. Control and placing feelings above sexuality indicate a mature degree of self-respect as well as a desire to find a "workable" relationship. Another way of looking at it is that sex is the final point in human development that permits an intense fusion.

Hypersexuality indicates a need for fusion that is not being met. Sex for sex's sake is indicative of an individual who denies his need to push people away by overcompensation with superficial closeness.

Devotees of the sexual revolution maintain that an individual who assumes a romantic attitude toward sexuality is "up tight." The sexual revolutionaries would have us believe that sex is *just* a natural biological function, as natural and, thus, unrestricted an act as eating or eliminating. But it is possible to survive without sex. Try that with eating or elimination.

However, the similarity is valid in another sense. The baby's earliest mechanism to reduce irritation is through the process of eating and elimination. Freud saw this removal of irritation as pleasurable for the infant. According to Freudian drive theories, the concept of pleasure and sexuality are interchangeable. This is an unfortunate choice in terminology. The feeding infant experiences pleasure as the hunger pain is removed. The organ systems involved with eating are the areas of the body that experience the pleasure (what really happens is that they experience a significant reduction of irritation).

Pleasure can be easily seen as a sexual concept. Reduction of irritation entropically cannot so easily be viewed this way. Most of us are unaware that our sexual behavior is motivated by a desire to reduce tension, not just sexual tension. If we view sex on a simplistic superficial level, we are not taking this into account. After all, how can we trust our deepest feelings or show our vulnerability to relative strangers or to people we know are only pursuing their own gratification. Promiscuous sex provides only self-contained release of tension.

The appeal of promiscuity at first may center upon a need to rebel against authority. Doing something that is questionable in society is appealing to the adolescent residuals of rebellion. However, its continued practice may also indicate that an individual is too frightened to let someone in.

One important symptom of self-containment is an obsessive need for orgasms. Masturbation is the bottom line of self-containment. As early as the Kinsey study, it was clear that everyone did it, and the rest probably lied about not doing it. When masturbation becomes obsessional, however, it is symptomatic of self-containment and a need to modulate hyperirritation internally. Masturbation is a very asexual act. It is the search for the soothing that mother should have provided, acted out through fantasies of her substitutes. It can easily be followed by anaclitic depressive reactions. Masturbation emphasizes, rather than reduces, isolation.

Extramarital sex and promiscuity are one step up from masturbation. You are almost certainly lying to yourself if you claim that you indulge in extramarital sex only because of a horrendous marriage and that you must seek a fusion outside of it. "My wife doesn't understand me" can be a double-edged lie. She may not, but you probably do not understand her and/or yourself either. How will casual sex with someone else help you understand either? If she does not understand you, perhaps her own needs to fuse cloud the issues. Perhaps, your needs to resist a fusion cloud your understanding.

If you really want the opportunity to fuse, you will either try to make your marriage work or get out of it. Then you can begin the search for someone to whom you can freely and openly fuse. But you are not going to find such a person on the next stool in a singles bar. Stop kidding yourself. The joke can be lethal in the long run.

I still obviously believe in motherhood and apple pie, and I even eat an occasional hot dog, nitrates and all. But when it comes to sex, my position is not based on morality or religion. Sexuality is one of the personality factors that contribute to an individual being precancerous or relatively immune. I advocate behavior that I believe will assist in developing immunity.

Prevention in Old Age
Old age is a high-risk time for cancer. Biologically, the degenera-

tion of cellular material, particular chromosomes and genetic materials, can obviously be said to be the cause. After all, a woman over thirty-five is at greater risk of giving birth to a genetically defective child than a twenty- or thirty-year-old. By age forty, the odds increase astronomically from the level at thirty-five. This is caused by the shifting of genetic material on the chromosomes. These translocations occur in the nucleus of the ovum. *Body* cells undergo the same type of degeneration. But this degeneration alone does not cause cancer. Age as an issue leads us back to the realm of external and internal carcinogens. People in the Crimea and Peru frequently live to be over 100 and are free of cancer. Aging is not an answer in itself.

One person works in an asbestos factory for a brief time and then finds new employment; another person works there for years. Statistically the long-time employee will run a much greater risk of cancer because the chemical irritation is cumulative. Over time it builds up.

Two recent medical school graduates decided to specialize in treating, and doing research on, cancer. After a couple of years, Dr. A. found dealing with such patients unbearably depressing, and he completed a residency in another specialty. Dr. B. developed all sorts of defenses to guard against the emotional irritation of his practice of oncology. He had a reputation for being detached from his patients' feelings but highly competent medically. Twenty-two years later Dr. B. died from a soft body-tissue cancer.

The emotional irritations caused by Dr. B.'s specialization were cumulative. Eventually, a translocation was reached and the land mine went off. The greater the depth of the placement, the more it is protected, the longer it may take for the cumulative effects of irritation to reach the site.

Whether the irritation is external (asbestos) or internal (the strain of being an oncologist), the effects will accumulate over time. It may take until the person is sixty-five or eighty-two.

Other aspects of aging and cancer are based upon the intangibles, the life events, and the feelings surrounding them. A sudden and abrupt ending to a significant emotional entropic system is a cause of cancer. The elderly have almost all lost close relationships through death. Previously I pointed out that we almost all know of someone who lost a spouse and then, almost immediately afterward, died of cancer. Losing parents correlates to cancer usually only for the very young. Losing a husband or wife, a child, a sibling, or even a job, correlates to cancer in adults. In a certain age category, a number of friends and relatives may die within close time intervals. If this happens to the young, as in war, the incidence of cancer is also elevated. Apparently, repeated losses can be biologically and emotionally intolerable for many individuals if they had the necessary infantile conditioning and translocations.

If you have a parent who has suffered a loss, there are important matters to consider to help assist in his or her survival. If the marital relationship was loving, people can adjust more easily. If it was not, guilt over the death of the spouse may be pronounced, and the need for punishment may be fulfilled by social isolation.

Help your parent to be in situations in which his or her contemporaries are present. If socializing is not permitted because of mourning traditions, then at least be there for the parent. Have the grandchildren accessible. And regardless of *your* feelings of disloyalty, encourage remarriage if at all feasible. Allow the parent appropriate time for grief but try to help to keep it from continuing for more than several months or half a year. Even that period of time is risky in that malignancies can develop in the bodily cauldron of internal carcinogens from the reaction to grief.

Another part of aging is the regressive aspect of growing old. The individual becomes more and more dependent as physical limitations set in. Older people need help but may be "too proud" to admit it. Often, they are too anaclitically depressed to admit it. A great deal of what is commonly referred to as senility has remarkable similarities to an autistic-stage regression. Grandpa may be lost in his own thoughts a great deal of the time. Grandma may not hear what is said more because of autistic residual than a hearing loss.

Thus, in old age, the accumulation of internal and external carcinogens may be coupled with a clear regression with marked autistic qualities. This corresponds to rapid cell growth at any age. The body is vulnerable to this growth—to cancer.

To help combat the autistic regression or residuals that are a necessary part of cancer development, always treat the elderly as older adults, not infants. Ask for their opinions, engage them in conversation and physical activity; have them do whatever they are capable of. *Do not infantilize the elderly.*

If they can work, they should be permitted and encouraged to do so. But they should not work in or around high chemical or physical carcinogen situations. No one should, but because of accumulations of carcinogens throughout the years, these irritants may be more hazardous with age. Work can help keep self-esteem high. Retirement for some people is equivalent to a death sentence.

Prevention During Stress

A few years ago, a new mental health field opened up. Originally, its purpose was to help top-level executives cope with "stress." Several years and lots of money later, it became obvious that top-level executives did not need, nor benefit significantly from, workshops or counseling on stress management. As a matter of fact, they seemed to thrive in high-stress environments. It was when the stress was removed that they became vulnerable to psychosomatic disorders.

Freud pointed out that preoccupation with external problems prevents the emergence of *internal* conflicts into the conscious mind. Top executives are frequently obsessive-compulsives who show signs of tunnel vision and total emersion in challenging problems. Perhaps their internal conflicts are far more dangerous than any external stress. The drive or need for success may be an enormous defensive structure, preventing the awareness of internal conflicts.

The dominant internal issue is anxiety. Anxiety is not based upon reality. It is a residual from the past that can permeate all aspects of the being. Perceptions become distorted, making situations that are not anxiety-provoking for most people highly threatening for the person suffering from chronic anxiety. Stress is not the equivalent of anxiety. It is based upon reality and would be perceived as threatening by almost anyone.

For a top-level executive, stress is manipulative; anxiety is not. Stress helps control anxiety for these people. As long as they can manipulate the variables adding up to stress, they love it; they thrive on it.

Seeking out stress is an anticancer defense for anyone whose anxiety reactions would produce overwhelming levels of internal carcinogens. As paradoxical as it may seem, stress apparently reduces the internal irritation of personalities prone to anxiety. But this stress is based upon matters that can be influenced by the individual. Top-level executives have a say in what stressful issues they will deal with. They make the decisions that result in success or failure for entire organizations. One would think this enormous responsibility would be extremely harmful. Not to these men and women. They have ways out that are directly under their control.

Carcinogenic stress occurs when an individual does not *need* stress as a defense or when the variables of stress are not under the victim's control. The stress-management people made an important discovery when they found that middle-management personnel were subject to all sorts of psychosomatic disorders, including cancer, when under stress. Why?

Middle-management personnel are in a position that can easily stimulate a reactivation of early conditioning for anxiety. For them, stress is frequently beyond their ability to manipulate the causes. They are at the mercy of both the top-level executives and the people they supervise. They must meet the needs of upper-level executives. In a sense they must "baby" them, be concerned for their feelings and reactions. But they must also meet the needs of the people working for them. At times middle management must choose between cajoling or coercing to get them to produce.

Middle-management personnel are the world of business's negotiators. They are the parents of both sides. Middle management is in a constant position of absorbing everybody's irritation. They are the implementers of the executive decisions. They are the recipients of negative morale, corporate malingering, or even unconscious and conscious sabotage. No one is there to absorb their irritation. Emotional entropy is not part of their work situation. Self-containment is far more likely to be the enforced psychological position. Stress for middle-management executives translates to coping with upsets and irritation from everyone. They cannot readily manipulate the variables or dissipate their own irritation.

Any stress that allows an individual to defend against anxiety and overwhelming internal carcinogens is anticancer. Any stress that places the individual in high-performance-anxiety situations in which the variables cannot be manipulated will produce high levels of internal carcinogens. Any stress that chronically places a person in the parental role while allowing for minimal dissipation of hyperirritation is highly carcinogenic. Middle-management personnel *must* turn to other life areas for fusion and emotional entropy. Unfortunately, their upsets frequently result in anaclitic depressions. They may take out their frustrations on the people who care most about them, making it very difficult for them to receive what they ideally need: verbal communication with a supportive loved one or, better yet, physical affection. A hug makes irritation leave the body as muscles relax and tensions fade. In the extreme, weakness may be felt as the entropic system is activated and working.

Three rules for the middle manager.

1. Don't be a stoic.
2. Don't be macho.
3. Don't be self-contained.

Prevention Through Exercise

I run 7-9 miles every evening after work. My dog runs alongside of me and is good quiet company. I notice some strange things happen when I run. My mind drifts through everything from Aristotle to business. It is strange that if I think of upsetting things when I am running, they don't seem so bad. I can't stay miserable about anything. When I think of bad things, I notice I exert myself a little bit more. It's as if I throw whatever it is off.

I notice my senses change. I know that sounds really way out, but listen to this. I figured this out because of my dog. On the way to the park where I run, my dog always urinates and defecates in the same area. Lots of other dogs use the same spot. I never notice the smell on the way to the park. I always notice it on the way back. I know you think it is because I'm breathing hard, but that's not the case. By the time I walk past that spot on my return, my senses really feel fine tuned. A rough towel after my shower can feel like sandpaper. I feel sexier and younger, also. I'm burning more calories, but I'm not as hungry. That I don't understand.

It has become like a drug. I feel really bummed out if, for some reason, I can't run. I'm nervous and tense. I even have to control snapping at people. I need the discharge running provides.

This man was one of a number of athletes I interviewed: runners, weightlifters, aerobic dancers, tennis players, and golfers. The joggers and weightlifters had the same reaction as the runner. This reaction may be anticancerous. Social contact, music, or competition prevents this phenomena.

As a person runs or lifts weights, the voluntary muscles are being used, with little mental involvement for successful completion of the task. Skill requirements are minimal. This permits the mental drifting that our runner describes. If your mind drifts like this while playing competitive sports or trying to keep in step with the aerobic dance class, you will lose miserably or stick out like a sore thumb. These activities require mental commitment. Running, bicycling, or weightlifting, in noncompetitive ways, do not. Simply stated, they permit a temporary regression to autism. As your mind drifts, you go in and out of this state. Coincidental with this regression is a powerful discharge of irritation through the voluntary muscles. Exercise on this kind of level may be preventive and possibly even somewhat curative with regard to cancer. The sensory vulnerabilities of infancy get reactivated. At the same time, an efficient dissipation of irritation is taking place emotionally and physiologically.

Studies indicate that people feel increased sexual desire after jogging or running. This may relate more to a desire for fusion than elevated hormone levels.

The entire process is a repetition from early infancy. Every day that exercise on this level takes place is another day of emotional reeducation if these guidelines are followed:

1. Exercise in isolation.

2. Do exercise that does not require concentration.

3. Avoid becoming competitive or training for competitive events.

4. Exercise without any distraction such as music or conversation.

If these principles are adhered to, this is perhaps the only individualized program of anticancer dissipation of irritation, but it is not an adequate anticancer program by itself. The necessary reconditioning for processing of irritation cannot occur through exercise alone. It is best to view exercise of this nature as a stopgap, almost emergency, measure. It should be part of a daily routine for high-carcinogenic-stress individuals, but it is equivalent to putting a dressing on an unsutured wound. It is not enough, but it is better than nothing.

Prevention of cancer, with the exception of exercise, is never a do-it-yourself proposition. "Do it yourself" is in itself a carcinogenic concept. Prevention of cancer requires fusion to another human being. It requires an emotional entropic system to dissipate or minimize irritation.

Cancer prevention is a "do-it-yourselves" proposition.

10

Spontaneous Cures: How They Relate to All Cancer Patients

A SEMANTIC DIFFICULTY arises in medicine and psychology when we discuss people who recover from cancer without medical or psychotherapeutic intervention. The usual medical term for such an occurrence is *spontaneous recovery*. In psychology, spontaneous recovery means the natural propensity to return to earlier patterns of conditioning. It is a return of previous learning after attempts (either conscious or unconscious) have been made to extinguish or turn off this learning.

If you have not ridden a bicycle in ten years, we might consider the ten-year interval as extinguishing the previous learning. The old adage that once you know how to ride you never forget is an example of spontaneous recovery. With very little effort, you fall back on the previous conditioning.

Psychologically, with cancer, spontaneous recovery would mean a return to the precancer symptoms or conditioning of emotional and physical responses to irritation, which would logically lead to another cancerous flare-up. Medical people call this a reoccurrence.

Therefore, for the sake of clarity, from this point onward, any reference to recovery from cancer with little or no medical or psychotherapeutic treatment will be referred to as a *spontaneous cure.*

Most of us have heard of cases of people with cancer who had little or no medical treatment, or whose treatment was stopped because the case was considered hopeless, and who ended up, nevertheless, apparently cured. Perhaps, they decided to trust in God rather than the medical establishment. Maybe the cancer was so advanced that the medical team felt that there was not enough likelihood of success to warrant the discomfort and dangers of the treatment. Perhaps, there were preexisting medical problems that precluded full-blown chemotherapy, radiation, or surgery. Whatever the reason for not receiving the full treatment or even any treatment, these people got better. Why? The experts appear to be baffled. "These things happen with cancer. We don't know why, but we do know it happens."

These cases require very careful investigation, both medically and psychologically, to shed some light upon the possible means for the prevention and cure of cancer. Who does not get cancer may be as important as who does. Who recovers and why is more important to investigate than who does not. Thus spontaneous cures should not be dismissed as just oddball medical curiosities. They may hold significant answers to which we have been paying little attention.

What we do observe in many, if not most, cancer patients is a medical process referred to as *cachexia.* This is the term for the sudden and shocking weight loss, weakness, excruciating pain, and general wasting away of the victim of this disorder. If you have ever cared for a terminally ill cancer patient you have seen these horrors and cannot easily forget their extremes. Again, many, if not most, terminal cancer patients die from the effects of cachexia rather than from the cancer itself. Pneumonia, failure of the heart or other organ systems, infections, and metabolic poisoning are perhaps the most common side effects of the *process* of cachexia.

This process has received little attention in the United States as opposed to the Soviet Union. We appear to be obsessed with the tumor and/or the neoplastic cells of cancer, when we should be considering cancer to be a *process*.

Cancer cells or a tumor drain nutrients and, thus, energy that would normally be distributed to the cells that are still doing their metabolic jobs. Cancer cells just reproduce and rob other cells of their life-support systems. Rob may be an understatement. They commit more of a monumental grand larceny—more like the Brink's job as opposed to shoplifting. The energy sources and reserves are depleted. Cachexia is the biological representation of the psychological phrase "eating yourself up alive." The process accelerates as the cancer cells reproduce and spread. Even if the victim could consume a great deal more food than usual, the tumor would drain the energy provided so that consumption becomes a losing battle. Typically, cachexia is somewhat accelerated by an aversion to food.*

Chemotherapy for most cancer results in nausea and diarrhea, thus causing loss of appetite and possibly hastening cachexia. The lining of the digestive tract is a rapidly reproducing tissue, and it is attacked by the poisons oriented toward any rapidly reproducing cells in the body. Cancer patients frequently stop almost all eating just as the cancer puts its most intense drain on the energy reserves of the body. The body starts to consume itself.

In every case of spontaneous cure that I have studied, the apparently doomed individual decided cachexia was not going to defeat him. In order to fight this process three elements were common to all.

---

*The act of eating has tremendous psychological value, however. For the cancer-ridden, it means accepting food from someone else in order to sustain life. This may be the value of coaxing the victim to keep eating regardless of discomfort. The patient must feel the caring of the nutrient provider.

1. Spontaneously cured patients forced themselves to eat.
2. They developed an obsessional drive for physical activity.
3. They resisted the regressive aspects of the disorder. In other words, they refused to stay alone, they occupied their minds, they fought depression with feelings of anger and determination to overcome the situation.

These spontaneously cured patients suffered from leukemia, pancreatic, lung, metastasized breast, and colorectal cancer. Medical experts agreed in all cases that these people were doomed. They all survived for longer than seven years.

Again, I wish to emphasize that modern medical techniques *should* be utilized whenever possible. At the least, they buy the cancer victim time. If that time is used for a thorough reconditioning, I believe the disorder can be reversed. The three steps common to all the spontaneously cured cancer victims should be followed by all cancer patients.

The first step is self-inflicted forced feeding. The patient must eat! And he must eat well-balanced meals to avoid carcinogenic irritation from eating one kind of food predominantly.

One person I spoke to explained that, at first, he threw up almost anything he ate. He would rest just long enough to end the urge to regurgitate and then eat some more. It was almost as if he were telling his stomach and esophagus that he was not going to let them give control to the cancer. Eventually the regurgitation stopped.

He followed none of the more learned approaches to nutrition and cancer. *He just plain ate!* He knew nothing of the technicalities of what to eat. He did know that if he gave in to the impulse to refuse food, he would die.

This man's cancer was pancreatic. Only two percent of pancreatic cancer victims live for five years after the diagnosis. His pancreatic cancer was diagnosed over twenty years ago!

For this man and for many others, the act of eating may be just as important as the nutrients consumed. In a weakened condition, the *apparently* terminal cancer victim is placed in a dependent role. He can certainly not prepare his own meals and may even have to be fed by someone. Being fed is a return to an early infantile position. Food represents the nurturance necessary to sustain life. It can thus be used as a means of communicating that the caring individual genuinely wants the cancerous individual to survive.

Spontaneously cured people eat. It is as simple as that.

They also move. Within the guidelines set by medical experts, if they have had any contact with them, or totally on their own, they get up and move. All of us who have convalesced from any illness know that if we stay in bed "resting" we really are staying in bed weakening.

Cancer puts a drain on one's energy reserves, so it would seem that conserving energy would be wise; but this does not seem to be the case. In all the spontaneous cures I have studied, the people moved.

Sometimes the efforts involved were staggering. Mrs. A. spent over an hour getting from her bedroom to the kitchen table. She associated eating in bed with dying in bed—her parents had died this way, and she was not going to let herself follow suit. After eating she would sit and talk with her family for a while and then spend the next hour working her way back to her bedroom.

This fifty-one-year-old woman had undergone many medical interventions. Surgically, she had had a radical mastectomy and a hysterectomy. Chemotherapy had been used but seemed only to weaken her. Radiation had also been used postoperatively, but the cancer kept spreading, in spite of all these efforts.

It was obvious to her that nothing was working and so she said, "No more." She took over. Her doctor told her family that at the most she had a year to live.

When she took charge, her condition appeared hopeless. She

had lost almost 20 percent of her body weight. Her skin was ashen, and her hair was almost completely gone. To keep her comfortable, her physician had prescribed pain medication, which left her feeling tired and out of touch with the world. Somehow she knew that this would destroy her if she continued it. On her own, she gradually withdrew from the pain medication. She grew to fear it as if it represented death itself. She may have been right.

If, as I have theorized, rapid cell reproduction is usually tied into an autistic regression, then pain medication may facilitate both. The weakness it causes will help keep the person spaced out and isolated. The use of depressants in cancer treatment promotes the emergence of autistic residuals while repeating the original conditioning of self-containment of irritation. These drugs do not encourage meaningful relating. Instead, the user looks, sounds, and, in almost all ways, acts extremely self-contained.*

Mrs. A. had welcomed the relief from pain, but the isolation and feeling of loss of control were terrifying. She knew they spelled doom, which gave her the strength to go against everyone's advice and gradually stop the pain drugs. In so doing, she may have affected the rate of cell reproduction. In other words, she may have interfered with the process of negative psychoplasia.

Her methods were based upon her unconscious awareness that she must do everything in total contradiction to what the cancer seemed to dictate. If she was nauseated, she ate anyway. If she was weak and tired, she forced herself to move. And the more she wanted to be left alone, the more she forced herself to relate to loved ones. She even explained to them that they should not fall

---

*If such medication seems necessary for the cancer patient, it should be used only to take the edge off pain, not remove all of it. Lamaze techniques of childbirth are based on a counterconditioning that shows remarkable ability to reduce pain. Similar techniques might be of use to the cancer patient. Perhaps most important, they would also require that the cancer victim relate to a coach, not a drug, for entropic removal of irritation (pain).

for her occasional nasty anger. She told them not to let themselves be pushed away, no matter what. Fortunately her family understood and tolerated the abuse she occasionally heaped on them.

She was a potter by avocation and had her wheel in the basement. She returned to this hobby as soon as she could, her only concession to her illness was to replace her pedaled wheel with an electric one. She could not work at her former speed, and what had taken two hours previously now required eight, but she stuck to it and created some beautiful pottery.

When she worked on her pottery, she planned the pieces as gifts for her family and friends. Thus, even though she was alone and isolated while pursuing her hobby, she had others in mind. She was also discharging irritation through her voluntary musculature.

Her cachexia stopped, and color returned to her skin. She began to look more as if one foot was out of the grave. Within a few months, she even looked as if both feet were out. There was no adequate medical explanation for her recovery, although her doctor sent her to a number of other specialists hoping to get one. They either suggested that perhaps the standard procedures had finally worked or they candidly admitted not knowing.

As a young graduate student, Professor W. contracted colon cancer. He had surgery performed as well as radiation and chemotherapy. When a reoccurrence of the disorder took place, he was told that nothing more could be done; but he was determined to defeat the cancer.

At about this time, he met a young woman whom he subsequently married. He was totally candid with her about the frightening facts of his cancer, but remarkably, she accepted him regardless and remained consistently supportive. When he became depressed and wanted to give up, his fiancée threatened to leave him if he did not continue his fight against cancer. The two of them researched nutrition, other medical techniques, and all sorts of alternative approaches and came to the conclusion that very little was making sense. They put together their own program for his rehabilitation. It included six to eight meals a day, plenty of movement and vigorous exercise, and a refusal to permit him to give up the music, art, and athletics that he had so much enjoyed in his precancerous existence. The program worked. Professor W. has been happily married for ten years now, is the father of two children, and has shown no signs of reoccurrence of cancer.

These people all recovered from cancer that "should" have killed them. They interfered with the psychological connections to the biological symptoms. They moved and discharged irritation through the voluntary musculature much in the manner of a newborn. They resisted the cancerous conditioning of refusing caring from others. They refused to permit the self-containment of the autistic stage. The negative psychoplasia was replaced with emotional entropy in which irritation was shared by the family. It is this interference with negative psychoplasia, along with reconditioning to process irritation entropically with others, that forms the basis of my recommended psychotherapeutic treatment plan.

All of these people have that certain spunk that makes them fight harder in the face of overwhelming odds. They are obsessional by nature and can thus persevere when many others would give up. They appear to almost enjoy their defiance of cancer! They are proud of their victories, and they are entitled to this pride.

As previously stated, the three steps work best in conjunction with medical treatment that buys time and/or cure in itself. My suggestions are not intended to assist the individual to deal with death and dying. Instead, this approach is designed to promote life. There is too much to accomplish and too little time to waste it on preparing for failure.

I definitely do not recommend any artificial imagery to encour-

166

age positive thinking. Such lying to oneself is a questionable expenditure of precious time and energy.

The next chapters deal with psychoanalytic treatment of the cancerous and precancerous individuals. We cannot correct translocations, but we can reeducate an individual to process internal and external irritation differently. When this happens, the body's defenses can stop fighting a losing battle and, instead, begin to win.

This chapter has shown that unique spontaneous cures can perhaps be explained within the confines of this theory. Spontaneous cure can be considered to be the bridge between prevention and psychotherapeutic treatment.

It is very important to remember that relying upon one's ability to achieve a spontaneous cure is hazardous and usually fatal. But, what we can learn from spontaneous cures can help in cancer treatment generally.

The following chapters are for both the professional and the layman. I apologize to the layman for some often necessary technical language in chapters 11 and 12. I do want to make the point that knowing a psychotherapeutic treatment plan will not affect anyone's ability to be treated. If this approach makes sense, perhaps, I can help motivate some victims and potential victims to consider such a course of action seriously. After all, why would anyone leave any reasonable stone unturned?

11

Treatment

We shall not cease from exploration and the end of all our explor-
ing will be to arrive where we started, and know the place for the
first time.

T. S. Eliot

IN A SENSE, DIAGNOSIS OF A precancerous personality or
even the awareness that one is treating a cancer patient is irrelevant. Any psychoanalysis that integrates learning theory and
drive theory should have as its aim the emotional reeducation of
the patient. A complete emotional reeducation for any patient
would imply that access to autistic-stage feelings has been
achieved. To do this the patient must regress through the anaclitic depression.

Our greatest ally in gaining access to the autistic stage for the
cancer patient is the *cancer itself*.

The Autistic-Stage Cancer Patient
With patients who do not respond to medical treatment, deterio-
ration is hastened by cachexia and medical intervention. Medica-

tion, pain, and fear have these patients in a thoroughly regressed state prior to their entering psychoanalytic treatment. Frequently, they are so weak and depleted that family and friends must help them into the analyst's office. Once there, they seem childlike in their lack of defensiveness. At the first session, they will show obvious signs of autistic-stage functioning. They will be in and out of awareness; perhaps, they will even doze and then suddenly awake. Their mental activity is far away; their eyes have a distant look. Perhaps, if they are very near death, they will report seeing spots or lines of light. There is a peacefulness and longing in their expression that hides the overwhelming irritations to which they have been subjected.

The analyst will usually see improvement in such patients almost immediately if he or she acts promptly and firmly. In order to comprehend this, a very simple fact must be remembered about the anaclitically depressed children René Spitz studied (see chapter 12). Their recovery was prompt if a loving mother returned before it was too late. The analyst who works to replicate a loving autistic-stage mother-baby fusion will be the mother returning in time.

With advanced cancer patients who are obviously functioning on an autistic-stage level, the analyst must intervene powerfully and convincingly to begin the recovery, as in the following example.

Analyst: If you agree to treatment now, I want you aware of the fact that you are stuck with me. There will be no leaving me until you are better. Any important decisions must be discussed here first.

Patient: OK (Smiling broadly)

Analyst: I'm taking over. You're mine now.

Patient: Everyone else was so "iffie." I know you won't believe this, but I feel better already.

Analyst: I'm glad, but there will be ups and downs. The impor-

tant thing to remember is that you and I will see this
through *together.*

Patient: (Laughing) I don't want to leave. When can I see you
again?

The analyst must immediately replicate the autistic-stage
mother-baby relationship. He should not be cautious or explora-
tory with such a patient. Such caution will place the analyst in
the same category as the other medical professionals who state
probabilities and statistics about survival. They say things that
make the patient aware of their fears and doubts as to whether he
will recover. They express hope reluctantly because of a desire to
avoid fake optimism. The analyst, on the other hand, cannot be
protecting himself from possible failure, considering the medical
realities of his new patient. Fusion must be worked toward
immediately; hope must be reinforced immediately; responsibility must be assumed immediately.

To anyone but an autistic-stage cancer patient facing death,
such an intervention would be viewed as absurd and bizarre. The
precancerous or optimistic cancer patient would think that such
an analyst has a problem with omnipotence and a desire to own a
condo on Mount Olympus. The cancer patient who has abandoned adult functioning under the pressure of the disorder and its
treatment will simply view the analyst as unlike everyone else.

For this desperately ill patient, there is no anaclitic depression
to be reached through psychoanalytic regression. It has been
reached and passed because of the severe effects of the cancer.
Years for building safety in the therapeutic relationship before
the patient will allow access to the autistic stage have been
brutally stripped away by the cancer. It is almost as if, in its
arrogance, the cancer has exposed its Achilles' heel.

The analyst must take this opportunity before it is too late. If
there is life and an ability to communicate in any manner, there is
hope!

After the initial contact during which the deeply regressed cancer patient is adopted, the analyst must periodically reinforce the maternal role:

Patient: Everyone is saying I'm looking better. I do feel better and I'm eating again. But they all think it is because the chemo is finally working. I don't think so. I haven't had any in months. When I tell them it is because I'm coming to you, they pooh-pooh it. And it gets me upset.

Analyst: They don't have to approve. You and I know what is going on. Everything between us is special. They wouldn't understand. Don't upset yourself trying to convince anyone. It's our secret.

Patient: They all think I'm talking to you to learn how to accept what's happening. When I say that I hear your voice saying that you will work with me only for a cure, they don't believe it. No one has said that to me in two years. When you first said it, it was like a breath of fresh air. It's like my mantra now. Only a cure, only a cure.

The patient continued to express a desire to get better. But at times, he was fusing by trying to please the analyst with claims of miraculous improvements, which represented a reverse entropy. So the analyst told him that he was expected to feel discomfort at times and even to be upset and depressed again. With this permission granted, the patient was able to report feeling overwhelming body sensations and being out of touch with his environment. When the analyst was aware of such stages, he had the patient close his eyes to facilitate the regression, and the autistic sensations became even more powerful.

The cancer patient should be instructed to use the couch as soon as possible. The eye contact is fusional in the original autistic stage. We have all witnessed the intensity of a mother and her baby's eyes meeting together in a fusional gaze. But eye contact for any adult, even an autistic-stage patient, can cause discomfort and confusion. The patient may feel embarrassed at being stared at or misunderstand the analyst's facial expression.*

In addition, although infants may experience fusion through eye contact, adults have had too many unpleasant experiences of being forced to look perceived tormentors in the eye for this to happen. Just recall your discomfort when a parent or teacher forced you not to look away while verbally attacking you.

Another reason I recommend the use of the couch is to facilitate repetition of bodily sensations of the newborn stage. The bodily position of the newborn is one of reclining and looking up. However, the analyst should instruct these reclining adults to close their eyes, which permits the patients to get lost in themselves. This is the nature of autism. Thus, closed eyes are the regressive partner of the reclining position.

As the patient goes deeper into the autistic state, he will report feeling strange bodily sensations. Extreme fluctuations may occur. For instance, the patient may report that his limbs feel heavy and then light, or perhaps, they tingle. Some patients say that they feel crazy at these times. They are correct in that they are passing through the developmental stage that relates to the psychotic defenses. Observation of the patient's movements is of utmost importance as he undergoes the reactivation of the neonatal stage. When he is experiencing hyperirritation, he will attempt to discharge it through fidgety movements. If this defense remains purely autistic, feet or hands may shake, arms or legs may move, knees may alternately be drawn up to a bent position. This is the newborn's means of discharge through the voluntary musculature. With the adult asutistic-stage cancer

---

*Freud eventually admitted he had patients use the couch to avoid eye contact, which he found intolerable. Interestingly, Freud died from cancer. He also was, in my opinion, anaclitically depressed. Eye contact would not have been his forte.

patient, this movement appears involuntary, but it is quite similar to that of the overstimulated newborn.

The patient may resort to higher-level defense if he is fluctuating between autism and symbiosis (awareness of an inside and an outside). In this case, movement will be the same; but in addition, the patient may intermittently cross his arms or legs; intertwine his fingers; or touch his abdomen, head, or chest.

In both instances, instruct the patient to remain still and do not permit him to hold onto himself. In other words do not permit a closed self-contained system. Taking this defense away will result in further verbal expression of primitive sensations.

The first time an analyst witnesses such a physical reaction is usually startling. He may fear the patient is evolving into permanent psychosis. In order to stop this phenomenon all one has to do is ask the patient several successive questions or instruct him to sit up. The reaction immediately disappears as the regression is abruptly terminated. But allow at least five minutes for the patient to compose himself before he leaves.

This state of hyperirritation provides the opportunity to recondition toward fusion. But the patient will not demonstrate these raw feelings unless the analyst is calm and dedicated to soothing. The patient always anticipates that the involuntary reactions of the analyst will be similar to the autonomic reactions of the maternal figure. He must feel secure to be able to tolerate the discomfort of the hyperirritated state in the presence of another person. The analyst should intervene minimally while the patient is primarily functioning on an autistic level, keeping in mind that the purpose is to establish the appropriate emotional entropy that should have been learned the first time around. Remain silent unless you are needed to foster the reeducation. Remember that you are dealing with a *totally* preverbal conditioning.

The analyst merely has to be there with a genuine desire to cure the patient. Remember, words do not matter to autistic-stage people (infants or adults). The tone and the feeling of a communication is, without a doubt, far more important than the content of what is said. At times words may actually cause an interference and be viewed as grating irritations to a patient at this stage. The analyst is there to meet the patient's emotional need; therefore, he should wait for the patient to speak first. If the patient is being asked to respond to the analyst, it is a reversal of emotional entropy. The analyst instructs the patient to speak at the beginning of treatment. That is all the instruction that is necessary. Merely saying, "Talk to me," is enough to establish whether the patient is resistant to communicating charged thoughts or feelings. But with an autistic-stage cancer patient, any words beyond those that contribute to the fusion are superfluous and potentially irritating.

As the patient begins to improve, the family of the patient may become a problem for the successful continuation of treatment. Just a few weeks ago, they were contemplating funeral plans. They had become afraid to hope; they have been preparing for the loss of a loved one. The physicians have made it clear that there is little, but more likely, no hope. They speak in terms of how much longer the loved one has left. They may even believe that the analyst is perpetrating a cruel hoax. They are afraid of what they do not understand. On occasion, family members will attack the treatment and become reluctant to cooperate.

Regardless of how tempting it would be to bring the family together to help manage such resistance, the analyst would be wise to exclude them. Any other person present when the patient and analyst are together will be viewed by the patient as an interference with the fusion. Any other person present will also interfere with the expression of autistic-stage sensations. It is also important not to see the family separately from the patient, for this could make the patient feel betrayed.

Keep the family away, and rely on the patient's urgent need for contact with the analyst to resolve family resistance to coopera-

175

tion. Even if the family is resistant, the patient's need will not be denied. Above all, the purity of the fusional relationship must be maintained.

For this reason, the analyst should not begin treating such patients unless he is as certain as possible that he will not have to leave the patient for at least several months. A vacation or even a medical emergency for the analyst could prove to be a separation of disastrous consequences. Plan as carefully as possible for such contingencies.

As the patient progresses through the autistic stage and into symbiosis (the beginning of object relations), he will not need the defense of the infantile or anaclitic depression. If the autistic-stage issues are dealt with to promote fusion, the patient will not have to defend against contact with the outside world since the analyst is viewed as safe to relate to. When the patient was hyperirritated in the treatment situation, the analyst was soothing and comforting. Emotional entropy dissipated the patient's irritations. The involuntary nervous system is being reconditioned to seek soothing and comfort from another human being The biochemistry that contributed to the activation of the unstable genetic material is being changed. The addiction to fight or flight chemical reactions is being cured. And the body's natural defenses are no longer fighting this inner-directed attack. Instead of chronic depletion by the cachexia, they can reconstitute themselves and help repair the previous damage.

The patient wants to rid himself of this ultimate irritation called cancer. If the mechanism is to permit the analyst to function as the absorbing early mother, the analyst will be subjected to emotional and, thus, biochemical irritation. He must therefore protect himself. He will be most fortunate if he has an anticancer marriage. He must have had a thorough, personal analysis. He must be innoculated prior to working with hyperirritated patients. In addition, no one should see more than one such patient a day. And a beginning patient may have to be seen twice a week.

The autistic-stage patient must also have access to the analyst via the phone at any time. Babies do wake up at 2 A.M. for a feeding! The analyst would be well-advised to plan mindless exercise activities for a time period immediately after these scheduled sessions. He should have no contact with his children and, perhaps, even other patients until he has dissipated the absorbed irritation.

Of utmost importance to the patient is to avoid specialists who primarily treat cancer patients. If the analyst sees many such hyperirritated patients, treatment cannot be successful. In the first place, his patients will most likely outlive him; and in the second place, he will be unable to do an adequate job.

Oncologists have a significantly higher cancer rate than physicians with any other specialty. Analysts who would *specialize* in treating cancers will probably wind up with an even higher cancer rate. In addition, the need to defend against being overwhelmed themselves will result in the analyst's resistance to absorbing irritation, which will then diminish his effectiveness with his cancer patients. Avoid specializing in cancer treatment.

The Optimistic Cancer Patient and the Precancerous Personality
It is paradoxical that the precancerous and optimistic cancer patient are much more difficult to treat than the extremely regressed patient. The dynamics of cancer are not an ally in fostering regression in these people. Instead, cancer conditioning functions as a fifth columnist fighting against a reconditioning. These patients are functioning on far more mature defensive levels than the person facing immediate death. It is these mature defenses that create obstacle after obstacle to the regressive process. It is these mature defenses that deny direct access to the autistic stage. Layer after layer of this onion must be peeled away to get to the center.

Going backward, or regression, is the mechanism that permits this access. The regression is facilitated by permitting and encouraging the patient to say whatever he wishes to communicate. The analyst's role is to accept unconditionally any and all communication, particularly that fraught with emotional significance. As the patient learns to trust the safety of the situation and the analyst, two things of great importance occur. The first is that the analyst comes to be seen as the parental figure who should have treated the patient in this fashion originally. The second is a desensitization of emotionally overwhelming conflicts.

As the patient is encouraged to say everything, the emotional impact of the past is greatly reduced. The analyst's acceptance of verbal communication replicates what should have transpired originally when the patient/child was overwhelmed with feeling. The state of being overwhelmed translates to biochemical reactions regardless of what developmental stage is dominant.

Whether the patient is an egocentric attention seeker or shy and withdrawn or somewhere in between, he will assume an omnipotent position. He may react to *anything* negative with a why-does-this-happen-to-me attitude. He uses his sense of omnipotence to maximize his upsets. After all, it only happens because of him. He feels the pressure of believing he should be able to do something about it. When he cannot, even though no one else could, he attacks himself.

The optimistic cancer patient can be recognized simply from his medical history of a malignancy. His prognosis is good, and he wishes typically to deny fears of the likelihood of reoccurrences.

For the precancerous personality, proper diagnosis is more difficult but just as important, for a premature termination of treatment may result in greater likelihood of the development of cancer. The following should be looked for:

1. A history of hypersensitivity to chemical and physical irritants

2. A heightened sensory sensitivity

3. A need to care for others while refusing to permit the reverse

4. An inability to relate in moments of hyperirritation.

5. An inability to tolerate closeness without conspicuous discomfort

With cancer patients who have experienced spontaneous cures without medical or psychoanalytical intervention, the cancer itself facilitated a regression to autism. And in all of these cases, there was "someone there" for the patient who got past the anaclitic depression and permitted a fusion. The analyst's task is to be that "someone there" as well as to help the patient regress through the anclitic depression to the autistic stage.

The task is a difficult one because the mature defenses of the precancerous and optimistic cancer patient are on the alert to prevent access to the autistic sensations. If this neonatal stage was the scene of a conditioning for later cancer, if it was the scene for conditioning of self-containment in the face of hyperirritation, why would anyone want to risk confronting the autistic-stage fears of marasmus that cancer delays. Perhaps the only thing that permits the patient to seek and stay in treatment is his rational denial of this fear of confronting these sensations. Moreover, it is these very sensations that he seeks relief from. The analyst is unconsciously viewed as an overwhelming other. *But until the patient approaches the anaclitic depression, he will feel it would be irrational to be frightened of the analyst or the analytic process. Thus, these more mature defenses, while establishing obstacles, at least permit the patient to stay in treatment.*

The analyst's task initially is to help the patient avoid direct confrontation of the autistic-stage feelings. He does this to prevent immediate termination of treatment.

For most patients with this diagnosis, initial treatment may be like treating anyone else. They may be anxious but pleasant as they test the waters. However, some of these patients may be reluctant, passively aggressive individuals for the first few meetings. If the analyst suggests that the patient tell him the story of his life, the patient may cover his entire fifty-two years in ten minutes and then not know what to talk about next. For a month or more, the patient may spend all his time objecting to being in the analyst's office. He will say that he does not feel comfortable with the treatment or that he does not believe in this stuff. If the analyst joins or reflects the patient's fears, the defenses may be suspended long enough for the patient to find out that he does not have to deal immediately with the fear of annihilation that he experienced as a newborn.

As treatment progresses, patients in both categories will report fears of exploding from overwhelming irritation. The cancer patient will express this in terms of fear of recurring cancer. The precancerous individual will describe feeling as if he will die from the continuation of such torment. The precancerous patient seems to know that he is at risk. He may even express a genuine chronic fear of cancer.

Telling a patient who has had cancer (or is precancerous) not to worry about his condition or situation is an attack on his defenses. The patient will feel, perhaps rightly so, that the analyst does not understand him. Going along with the patient's fears allows the patient the opportunity to see the analyst as similar to himself. If the analyst wishes to lessen the impact of worry he should tell the patient that he can't be expected to do anything else but worry and that perhaps he does not worry enough. This provides for the feeding of the conditioned response of worrying and, thus, temporary relief.

The analyst may have to interpret a resistance to permit the patient the opportunity to be aware of his investment in being irritated. This frequently makes so much sense to the adult parts of these patients that it helps reinforce the continuation of treatment.

In general the treatment for the optimistic cancer patient and the precancer patient is the same as for anyone else. The analyst works to foster a relationship that permits the verbal expression of any and all thoughts and feelings. However, the more powerful the emotional impact of what is being said is, the closer one gets to the anaclitic depression and, thus, the autistic stage.

One patient found it far safer to talk about his medical treatment and its side effects than about his feelings and human relationships.

Patient: I don't want to come here any longer. It's not going to help.

Analyst: That may be true, but how do you know that already?

Patient: I just feel that way. This talking isn't going to do any good.

Analyst: You're probably right that talking about your cancer isn't going to do any good. We both know it's terrifying and depressing. What more can be said about it?

Patient: Nothing, you're right. But how will talking about anything make any difference?

Analyst: It might not, and it's already been three sessions.

Patient: Okay, I get the message. But each time I am preparing to come here, I feel as if my body is suddenly empty inside. The only other times I felt that way was when I first was told I had cancer and when they put me in that huge radiation machine.

Analyst: Why do you insist upon discussing cancer and how terrifying it can be? That's a fact we are both aware of.

Patient: You're right. This morning I couldn't eat a thing. I felt really nauseated. But the doctor said that will subside in time. All right, no more cancer. How come I can't stop with it here and at other times I can't mention it?

Analyst: Is it possible that you already know it's okay to say anything here?

Patient: Yes, but I can't stop talking about cancer here, and I can't even tolerate hearing the word anywhere else.

Analyst: Then you had better tell me any thoughts or feelings you have ever had in regard to cancer. (The analyst is deliberately joining the resistance of only being able to talk of cancer as a means of avoiding feelings. The patient no longer has to maintain this obsession.)

Patient: When I first got married, my mother died of cancer. She was very sick for almost a year with lung cancer. She died a month after I got married.

Analyst: Tell me about her. What was she like?

Patient: She was short and sort of chunky until she got sick. She was always there when I needed her. I wouldn't call her affectionate but she wasn't an iceberg either. If I needed her, she was there for me.

The patient continued a moving description of a young mother who took care of illness, injuries, and failures. But it was later revealed that she was incapable of giving any physical affection and never came near unconditional love. Gradually the patient came to realize painfully that he always pushed others away and felt disgust at any demonstration of physical closeness.

In order to keep an optimistic patient or precancerous individual in treatment long enough to make any difference in terms of reconditioning, a full knowledge of the technique of psychological reflection is necessary. Confrontive, insightful, or interpretative approaches are contraindicated. Anyone who doubts this should try talking a paranoid schizophrenic out of his delusions sometime. He will either attack or withdraw into himself.

The essence of reflective psychological technique is to strengthen defenses enough so that the patient is no longer invested in their maintenance. This is accomplished through the analyst's providing of a mirror of the patient's emotional state. At the same time that the defenses are being strengthened, the patient learns to perceive the analyst as being just like himself. Eventually he views the analyst as an extension of his own being. (Remember mother-baby bonding, which also lacks boundaries of the self.)

This eventually will permit the safety to allow a regression to the anaclitic depression. After the patient passes through the anaclitic depression, which will be discussed in the next chapter, arrival at the autistic stage can be recognized from the feelings that the patient will describe: drifting, strange bodily sensations; oceanic feelings; heaviness in different parts of the body; tingling sensations in the limbs, particularly fingers and toes; the sensation of floating around the room; dizziness; and so forth. It is the same as the experience of the originally autistic-stage cancer patient, that is, the one facing death in the near future. The patient finds this frightening because there is no conscious cause or explanation for these sensations.

Again, these patients will now also feel that they are going insane, and the analyst should encourage them to feel just that. The analyst must let the patient know that the analytic session is a safe place to experience such powerful feelings and that no explanation or excuse is necessary. Feelings and thoughts are just there, no matter how extreme. It is what one does with them that counts. No one has ever been confined in a psychiatric hospital for feeling crazy. It is necessary to act crazy first. Patients need to be reassured about this as they experience such intense feelings.

Analysts need to be reassured of it, also. The greater the capacity the analyst has to accept his own feelings, the greater the capacity to tolerate the patient's intense feelings.

If treatment fails, it may very well be because of the human inadequacy of the analyst. The powerful feelings that all cancer patients and precancerous personalities can induce are intolerable for the unanalyzed practitioner. At times they are barely tolerable for the most aware analyst. The analyst may come to experience various feelings that the patient's parenting agent felt during different stages of his development. These feelings may prevent a desire for fusion on the *analyst's* part. The analyst may periodically be detached, irritated, or anxious. The patient is experiencing similar feelings. As the analyst works to control his own level of irritation, he may be unconsciously working to stifle the expression of the patient's irritations.

At times it is reasonable to assume that the analyst may be replicating the mother's periodic inability to fuse with the infant during the autistic stage. At other times during the treatment, the analyst may experience other feelings the actual mother had. If the patient is being both provocative and defiant, it is safe to speculate that the analyst is experiencing the feelings of parenting a toddler through the "terrible twos" or a teenager through the autistic residuals of adolescence. If the practitioner yields to the desire to shut the kid up, he will confirm the original toxic learning and harm the patient.

The outbursts of the autistic-level patient may be whimpers or shouts with no *rational* explanation behind them. The analyst may feel that this is an intolerable amount of abuse to endure and work to cut off its expression. Although the patient's rage is merely a demonstration of infantile hyperirritation, if the analyst loses sight of this, he will feel attacked and injured by it. This will leave the patient with no alternative but to return to a self-contained emotional entropy. The analyst is, thus, replicating the original toxic response of the mother.

The entire purpose of such an analysis is to recondition the processing or irritation that originally occurred in the autistic stage. The analyst must be placed in the early maternal role in order to accomplish this. This transference of an earlier relationship onto the present therapeutic one is a natural phenomenon. All the analyst has to do to accomplish the development of such a relationship is to avoid getting in the way of its natural evolution. We all respond to life's stimulation based upon previous conditioning.

When the autistic-stage issues are dealt with, this surrogate mother will be viewed as the original inconsistent maternal figure. If the baby was irritated then, the patient will be irritated now. *The irritation that was added to the preexisting irritation was*

184

the first emotional and biological conditioning of this person. Cancer is the fulfillment of this conditioning. Thus, the surrogate, the analyst, is viewed as the ultimate irritator, the cancer itself!

No artificial symbols are needed. The patient is plagued by symbols of cancer while asleep and awake. The analyst is the most workable symbol. This is because of the analyst's ability to change the response. The analyst does not have to add irritation to the system at the patient's vulnerable points. The analyst can soothe and comfort in the way an ideal mother should have behaved. But this soothing and comforting will not result in a reconditioning unless the autistic-stage issues are reached and the analyst comes to be viewed as the overwhelming irritator, the cancer or predisposition for it.

Once the hyperirritations of the autistic stage are achieved, the analyst and patient will perhaps go through periods of what appear to be rage and love (but is more accurately called hyperirritation and homeostasis) that make both feel fused to the other. The feelings on both sides of the couch may be peaceful or agitated, but they are conspicuously thoughtless. Cognition may be absent in the analyst at this point. How then can he know what to do or say? The truth, perhaps, is that after the rage has been expressed, he does not have to know. His positive feelings for the patient are the only guidelines he needs.

The one exception to this is the patient's desire for physical contact. The analytic rule of no physical contact must be maintained. More mature feelings can easily return, and physical contact can be treatment destructive as the therapeutic relationship rapidly leaves autism and seeks eroticism. Both the analyst and the patient may have powerful compulsive feelings to hold and be held. This must be refused, or the regression may be rapidly reversed.

It is the resolution of the expression of rage (hyperirritation) that is ultimately the path to autistic fusion. If this does not happen, then regression will be halted due to the patient's feeling a lack of safety in the relationship. The patient's desire to destroy the analyst will then be projected, and fear will preclude the expression of anger and dissatisfaction.

Many analysts probably experience an autistic fusion with patients while not recognizing it as such. In response to rage directed at them, they may have extremely powerful feelings of wanting to comfort and soothe the patient. If the opposite reaction occurs, however, the analyst must explore his reactions. If the analyst cannot comfortably love the patient at this point, the analyst had best avoid autistic issues with all patients. He himself needs to experience the correction of his neonatal defense system. If he does not, the dangers to the analyst and the patient may be greatly increased.

If the analyst insists upon not permitting self-containment and if he is dedicated to the survival of his patient, he may be working toward fusion without any conscious intent. But being unaware is a dangerous state for both the analyst and the patient, who cannot be expected to be aware of anything but feelings during autistic regression. Proper care for the patient rests in the analyst's hands. It is the same relationship as between babies and mothers. It is not the baby's responsibility to know anything. The analyst must take all the responsibility on his own shoulders. This is as it should be.

Group therapy or analysis for optimistic cancer patients or precancerous patients is contraindicated. It is altogether impossible for autistic-level cancer patients. Dealing with superficialities in a group will have little or no beneficial effect. If causal issues are dealt with in a group setting, there is a serious risk of repeating the original toxic conditioning, particularly if one patient ascribes the surrogate maternal role to another group member. No one who is unprepared can be expected to respond therapeutically to another's vigorous and, perhaps, bizarre expression of hyperirritation. Patients who are themselves emotionally and biologically undergoing infantile hyperirritation cannot possibly react appropriately to another patient. This type of therapy actually produces a group of upset babies.

On a superficial level, group therapy is fine for life-management problems. But no one can be expected to suspend enough defenses to express openly the strange and frightening feelings of autism in a group setting, nor would it be possible for a group leader to deal with such feelings appropriately.

Imminent Death and Resistance to Autism

There will be many people who will resist autism until death has almost claimed them. From apparently mature but irritated levels of functioning, they will suddenly enter a comalike sleep and expire. They are the individuals maintaining the anaclitic depressive position up to the very end. They push away and get others to leave them in isolation. The next chapter is largely devoted to them as it addresses the management of the anaclitic depression. At this point, I would just like to present a case that illustrates the use of reflective psychoanalytic techniques in gaining access to the autistic stage.

A student of mine was involved in the treatment of an eighty-two-year-old woman who was suffering from metastasized cancer, which had originated in her breast. The student was a nurse on the medical team, which had decided to treat only the patient's pain since she was now too weak and the cancer had spread too far to do anything else. The nurse received permission to attempt psychotherapeutic treatment, claiming that all she wanted to do was offer help in preparing the woman for death.

When the nurse first entered the patient's room, she saw a small, frail, emaciated looking older woman in a slightly raised bed. Her food tray was untouched. The staff had reported that Mrs. K., a widow with no visitors, only occasionally drank some water. Cachexia had apparently already overwhelmed her system. Her skin was pale, the dull color of the victims of starvation.

Student analyst: Do you mind if I come in here and hide out for a while? (Exactly what Mrs. K. was doing.)

Patient: (A grunt)

Student analyst: (Taking off her nurse's hat and putting her feet up on the window sill) I can't take it any longer, all the sickness, the misery. I hate being a nurse. If I go out into the hallway, they will make me do some more work. I just want to hide. I can't go on with this anymore.

Patient: Why are you bothering me with this?

Student analyst: The others told me that I wouldn't be disturbed in your room. They said you almost never talk and that you get almost no visitors. That sounds perfect to me. I need a place where I won't be disturbed. Do you mind if I switch on the radio?

Patient: (Angrily) Yes, I mind! What do you mean using my room as a hangout? Get out of here right now or I will report you. I am very sick and just want to be left alone.

Student analyst: I just want to be left alone, also. Face it, no one will bother to check up on you for at least a half hour, maybe longer.

Patient: (Shouting) Get out of here. Who are you? Why are you bothering me? What kind of nurse, a person, are you? You are not fit to be a nurse! Now get out or I'll have you fired!

Student analyst: Well, then, hit the buzzer and turn me in. I'm not moving. I am the worst nurse you ever met, and I can't stand being any kind of nurse. So go ahead, hit the buzzer.

Patient: I can't reach it. Hand it to me you young bitch!

Student analyst: Get it yourself or just be quiet.

This sort of thing went on for several more days. Finally, the patient began to give up her depression.

Patient: (Looking more alert and even somewhat groomed) It's you again. Can't you find some dying child to harass? Maybe a mother whose kid was just born with no arms? Just leave me alone.

Student analyst: Listen, I know an easy setup when I see it, and you are it. You still don't talk to anyone except to complain about me. They don't care. They even think you're lying. I've got them convinced.

Patient: You're a sadistic bitch! (With a slight smile) Would you just hand me that cup over there on the shelf?

Student analyst: Get it yourself. I'm only here to goof off, not to work.

Patient: You're a monster. I hate you with every ounce of strength in me.

Student analyst: That isn't much now is it.

Patient: (Crying) I'm so scared. Please stop torturing me. I need someone to care about me. It's crazy, but I know that someone is you. (Crying uncontrollably)

Student analyst: You're right. That someone is me. We'll see this through together.

Patient: I really need you. You're such a bitch, and I really need you. I must be crazy.

The patient turned eighty-five last year. Her weight gain is now actually a problem. She has to cut back on how much she eats. As far as the medical team is concerned, no cancer is presently observable. This case not only demonstrates that fusion can be achieved even with a patient who desperately works to push away but, also, how therapeutic emotional entropy can be. It is but one of many cases that turned around at stages that seemed utterly hopeless.

Most important, this woman's situation shows how immediately accessible autism is when the anaclitic depression is present. The immediacy of death strips away the defenses that conceal the infantile feelings.

In summary, the only patients who do not require a resolution of the anaclitic depression are those so thoroughly regressed by the effects of cancer and the treatment for it that they are already functioning on an autistic level prior to entering analysis. They have no place else to regress to. The optimistic cancer patient and the precancerous individual are far from an intense anaclitic depression. However, residuals of it and the autistic stage can be observed in their inadequate ability to relate to others. This inadequacy is in not being able to accept love and caring. The cancer patient who is at the anaclitic depression level of functioning will, as with the first category, be confronting death. But this individual unconsciusly knows that autism represents the ultimate vulnerability. The desperation in pushing away is remarkable. The next chapter deals with this problem of managing this pushing away. All three categories share aspects of autism and the anaclitic depression. The predominance of one level or the other determines the treatment plan. They must all undergo an autistic reconditioning.

For all three categories discussed, what is curative is the emotional reeducation that takes place through fusion and emotional entropy. Involuntary areas of the nervous system are harnessed to support life rather than kill the patient. The processing of irritation is relearned to permit the individual to minimize internal carcinogens while no longer seeking external ones. The immune system can now work to aid in recovery rather than merely containing the effects of internal irritants.

12

Infantile Depression

IT WAS IN 1947, IN POSTWAR Switzerland, that René Spitz, M.D., first studied foundling-home infants. His book *The First Year of Life* attempted to answer some of the questions about psychologically deviant development in babies. The study was limited in that the infants observed were all chronologically past the autistic stage. The babies studied had been separated from their mothers somewhat after this stage. Their physical needs were well provided for by nuns, who performed their caring tasks efficiently, but the babies' emotional needs were all but ignored. There was no time for play or cuddling. There was no understanding of the significance of the baby's need to fuse. (Recent studies in hospital units for the newborn show that even premature babies who are held and talked to will take more nourishment per feeding session than if they are just fed "efficiently.")

Of 123 children observed by Spitz, 19 of his original subjects displayed a clear-cut syndrome, which Spitz referred to as *anaclitic depression*. In the second half of their brief lives, these babies changed from relatively happy individuals to weepy, withdrawn, immobile creatures, who even averted their faces to avoid interaction with anyone. If the approach of an outsider was "insistant," that is, the outsider would not be put off by the

baby's avoidance mechanisms, crying and occasionally screaming would follow. The babies lost weight. Insomnia was so bad
that the babies had to be separated to prevent them from keeping
each other awake. They were all prone to colds.

After three months of a loveless environment, the pathetic
weepiness subsided. It was replaced by a "sort of frozen rigidity of
expression." Spitz describes the babies as lying or sitting with
"wide-open, expressionless eyes, frozen immobile face, and a
faraway look, as if in a daze, apparently not seeing what went on
around them." The babies were regressing to the autistic stage,
characterized by a self-contained entropic system. They were
going back to the first emotional stage of life.

They had all been separated from their mothers between the
sixth and eighth month of life for a three-month period. If the
mother returned after the three-month period but prior to the end
of the fifth month, most children recovered. Spitz states that "in
anaclitic depression, recovery is prompt when the love object is
returned to the child within a period of three to five months. If
there are any emotional disturbances of lasting consequence,
these are not readily apparent at the time." Spitz speculated,
however, that although he was not able to determine consequences, in the long run, he felt "scars" would show up later in
life.

If similar emotional conditions surround any newborn, the
scars that will show up later in life are *cancers*.

After the fifth month of separation from the mother, symptoms
become even more severe. The prognosis is poor. The anaclitic-
depressive reaction is not comparable to adult depression, which
is viewed by Spitz as the result of a "sadistically cruel superego
under whose relentless persecution the ego breaks down." At this
stage in infancy, not even the precursors of guilt and conscience
are present.

Spitz observed that babies whose early relationships with their
mothers were negative did not experience the same severity of

suffering in the anaclitic depression as did the babies who had had positive maternal influences. Infants with a background of "bad" mothering were seen as having experienced relatively negative nurturing. Spitz described these babies as suffering from "mild depression" and believed that the syndrome masked deviant problems of a qualitative nature. Perhaps, what Spitz was observing was a *fixation* at the autistic stage. The babies from negative backgrounds would not have entered a well-defined symbiosis with another person. At the least, a predominance of autistic residuals would characterize the immature personalities.

Spitz felt that good mothering prior to separation resulted in a powerful trauma to the abandoned infant, with severe consequences. In other words, it was more upsetting to dissolve a viable entropic system than a weak, negative one.

The anaclitic depression that Spitz described may be viewed as the first interstage regression in life. The baby has entered a symbiosis, which is the next stage up from autism, with the mother. The baby is still powerfully attached to the mother but is beginning to see her as something outside of himself when the symbiosis is abruptly suspended. The child has no choice but to attach his drives onto something. If the self is all that is available, the attachment is self-contained—there is a clear return to the self-contained entropy of a negative autistic experience.

What Spitz observed was a tremendous shift of entropy back to the self-contained system of an emotionally neglected newborn. *In the babies who were already emotionally neglected or abused, there was little shift of entropic factors.* Some irritation had to be siphoned off, but to a large extent irritation remained lodged within the body and mind of the baby. Damage had already begun in terms of negative *emotional* conditioning. Spitz was observing *prepsychotic* etiology (causation) in these "mildly depressed" infants.

The anaclitic depression is nothing more than regression to

autism from a symbiotic stage. Thus, the anaclitic depression is an autistic self-contained entropic system. It is characterized by an autistic management of emotionality being coupled with the developing physical and mental abilities of the symbiotic stage. The baby in symbiosis can better communicate his emotional state; thought is more clearly evolving. When these factors are united with the autistic elements, the communication of self-containment is more easily discerned. The baby averts his eyes and face, cries, and even screams when contact is forced. He pushes away rigidly when held. Spitz's descriptions of the babies are overwhelmingly powerful. The terror and anguish in confronting the assumed aggressive maternal agent is enormous. These autistic residuals can remain throughout life.

The anaclitic depression may be the key to severe psychosomatic disorders. Cancer, being the most primitive biological disorder, demonstrates this in the most powerful way. To appreciate its significance, let me offer an analogy. When we approach birds on a beach, deer in a country setting, or even a strange dog on a street, they all have the same reaction. Up to a certain predetermined distance they will permit our approach. As soon as we step over the line, they flee or at least back up to reestablish that original distance. On occasion they may even make threatening gestures. The anaclitic depression is this mechanism on a human level. The human infant cannot flee and the human adult chooses not to because maturity has taught his intellect that there is no *real* danger. But his feelings may be the same as the sandpiper's or the deer's. (Equivalent brain areas relate to this phenomenon in both the human and the lower animal world.) However, with this inability for flight or fight (we know what a cornered animal can be like), we are left to express the anaclitic depression in terms of our biochemical reaction and personality traits (as previously described).

Foresters have told me that forcing deer into crowded, enclosed areas results in high mortality rates. When I asked what they died from, the reply was that "cancer frequently seemed to be the culprit."

With patience and caring, we can train birds and other wild animals to allow us to be comfortably close. We can get past the primitive brain functions of lower animals just through repetitive conditioning. Man is harder to deal with because of his intelligence. But once more advanced defenses (intelligence) are suspended, we gain access to these primitive brain functions.

The anaclitic depression is one of the first clear symptoms of a precancerous personality. Later in life, difficulty in accepting love and in feeling connected with others may add to a precancerous diagnosis. The precancerous person will push others away either subtly or overtly. He will be hypersensitive to irritation or impingements from others. Psychosexual errogenous zones, instead of being employed as centers of pleasure, will function as repositories of irritation within his self-contained entropic system and, thus, be highly vulnerable to cancer.

Whatever his defenses are, they will be used to reinforce his original autistic conditioning, which is thus encapsulated within the defenses of more mature levels of development. It is only when this encapsulation is removed and the autism is laid bare that the basic drives are accessible for emotional reeducation through conditioning toward fusion. Prior to this, the analyst will be dealing with more advanced levels of defense. It is only when all the defenses are temporarily suspended that the correction of the negative entropic system can occur. It is only at this point that the basic drives (hyperirritation and homeostasis) can exist simultaneously for the patient through a fusion with the analyst.

It is this fusion, which was discussed earlier, that provides the precancer or cancer patient with the opportunity to experience both irritation and homeostasis within a singular system. Thus, when the analyst can be viewed as the source of hyperirritation (the cancer), the signal for fusion is present. If the analyst responds with a communication of caring in the face of irritation, corrective reconditioning will be taking place. If the fusion is based upon the analyst's adding irritation to the patient's irritation, then this union will be carcinogenic.

Suspension of the defenses against the expression of autistic irritation within the therapeutic relationship is the goal of the first step in treatment. At each developmental level, various defenses will be activated to prevent autistic-stage annihilation (marasmus). The patient's anticipation is that his expression of irritation will be met with the analyst's irritation. Prior to access to the basic drives, the patient must learn through a suspension of more advanced stages of defenses that the expression of rage within the analysis will result in acceptance of his feelings by the analyst. If this does not occur, the patient will become guarded. Superficial granting of permission to express rage will not work. Superficial explanation of the defense and its causal factors will not work. What does work is reflective psychoanalytic techniques properly administered at the correct times.

Suspicion of the defenses of the anaclitic depression requires an understanding of the diagnosis and dynamics. The anaclitic depression is the last line of defense the cancer patient has prior to reaching the rawness of autistic feelings or prior to death. Elisabeth Kubler-Ross in *On Death and Dying* points out that the more advanced stages of defense precede the depressive stage prior to the acceptance of death. It is my contention that after the other defenses are suspended, after the anaclitic depression is suspended, the patient has the opportunity to deal with *the acceptance of life!* Death will be inevitable if the irritation and homeostasis are not reconditioned into a fused state. The depression that Kubler-Ross observed is a signal for optimism that perhaps something can be done. Kubler-Ross's depressive stage is an *adult* depression. Her clinical error is in not connecting *acceptance* to the anaclitic depression. There is overlap, but the quiet, sedate, and "peaceful" person, perhaps, dying from cancer, may be turning away from others in an anaclitic depressive reaction.

196

The analyst must take into account the nature of the defenses observed by Spitz in the anaclitically depressed infants. They turn away; they reject, become rigid, scream, and cry pathetically to get the maternal agent to put them down. The analyst must understand any resentment of attack that this behavior generates in him. If he can remember that he is dealing with a terrified baby who believes he is going to be killed, then the analyst cannot, and will not, put the baby down! He will hold on long enough to allow the rigidity to subside. He will gently insist upon being connected and involved in spite of all the patient's need for "space," distance, and isolation. *He will not put the baby down!*

Defenses against the therapeutic relationship and in the service of depression will manifest themselves in many ways, but the predominant defense will be to exclude the analyst. The patient will talk of other people in his life, significantly excluding this surrogate mother.

Patient: I was thinking about all the men I've known in my life who really amounted to nothing, yet I continued the relationships until I got them to leave.

Analyst: What did these men have that I don't have?

Patient: They were bastards. Since my divorce, I've known only bastards. My ex-husband is a bastard.

Analyst: What did they have that I don't?

Patient: You're not a bastard. You're nice to me.

Analyst: Are you saying you'd be more involved in a relationship with me if I were a bastard?

Patient: I guess that's what happened. First, it was my husband, and now, Peter has been the worst yet. I still can't end it. I'm afraid to tell him how sick the doctors say I really am. He'd cut out on me. [The patient continued for ten minutes complaining about the sadistic men with whom she had had relationships.]

Analyst: What would it take for you to be interested in me?

197

Patient: Why do you keep butting in? You're not my type and you never will be.

Analyst: You'd better help me to be your type because when it comes down to it, it's just you and me anyway.

Patient: Then I'm in a lot of trouble.

Analyst: Is this your first awareness of being in a lot of trouble? You have cancer. Can there be more trouble?

Patient: Why do you do this to me? You're a sadistic, egocentric son of a bitch. You think you're the only one who can help. What about my chemotherapist and the surgeon and all of them?

Analyst: When it comes down to it, it's just you and me.

Patient: Then what happens if something happens to you? [Negative wish for the analyst to die.]

Analyst: You'd better hope nothing does. [A deliberate replication of the earliest autistic relationship.]

Patient: You know, sometimes, I don't know if you're for real, but I do know how much I hate you. I just want to be left alone. I want you to stop suffocating me. Leave me alone!

Analyst: Give it up. You know I'll never leave you alone. You're stuck with me. You can't leave and I can't go. We have to see this through.

Patient: I know I can't quit, but I feel like I really want to when you pull this shit! It's not fair. I'm a prisoner.

Analyst: You're right. It's not fair. [Unconsciously addressing the cancerous aspects of the therapeutic relationship.] What does that have to do with anything?

Patient: [In a rage] I hate you. I really hate you. I hate you so much! [Crying] Please be nice to me. Stop doing this. I want you to care about me. [She was sobbing uncontrollably at this point.]

Analyst: When you can express yourself this honestly, anyone, even I, could have loving, caring feelings about you. [Said very gently]

198

Patient: I don't understand what is happening.
Analyst: You don't have to.

This was not the final resolution of the anaclitic depression, but it was a beginning. The patient, a forty-two-year-old woman, oscillated from the depressive need for isolation to the expression of raw autistic feelings. She frequently reported powerful bodily sensations once the anaclitic depression was being dealt with. In some sessions, all the analyst did was to repeat the patient's communications back to her. This was usually the precursor to the baby's need to push away actively. The analyst's response would be to hang on verbally and then offer communications of caring. Once the patient (baby) realized she could not succeed in overpowering the analyst (mother) she was able to relinquish the rigid rejection and accept love. One suspension of the anaclitic depression is not enough. Many repetitions will have to occur.

It is very important not to use psychological reflection of this resistance, which would only help maintain the defense when the object is to suspend it to allow brief doses of love into the system.

Overwhelming doses of positive regard (love, affection, understanding) are also contraindicated. One does not feed a victim of starvation a ten-course meal. The intake must be gradual and carefully metered or the very nurturance being offered may kill. When appropriately done, with each additional input of caring from the analyst in the face of the patient's irritation within the therapeutic relationship, autistic-level conditioning is being replaced by new life-supporting structures.

Misdiagnosis of the anaclitic depression can lead to further internalization and exacerbation of the precancerous or cancerous conditioning. The difficulty is to differentiate between depressive reactions on a more mature level and the anaclitic depression. The person suffering from a mature depression will be disturbed by severe feelings of guilt and castration fears. The more advanced stages of defense observed by Kubler-Ross, such as denial, bargaining, and anger, are all permeated with elements of this depression. The person is either fleeing from despondent feelings or he is using their components to lessen the impact. Making a deal with God to prevent death indicates the need to utilize guilt to lessen feelings of total depression.

The symbolic castration aspects of surgery and other medical techniques also serve to assist in the development of this more mature depression. After disfigurement the patient feels that certainly enough of a price in suffering has been paid. He may react as if he is almost pleased, without tremendous feelings of loss for the missing body part because the mastectomy or colostomy means he will survive. The depressive reaction to this symbolic castration has little connection to the anaclitic depression.

Patients report feelings of optimism if the surgery was a "success." They feel that if one suffers enough, gives up enough, endures enough, then he deserves to be rewarded with a "cure." The patient will either see himself or God as the omnipotent entity in this cruel bartering.

For far too many, however, the cruelty does not stop with the offering of sacrifices. The depression that follows may be anaclitic in nature. It does not appeal in any way to adult logic and is our medium of passage into the realm of autistic-drive reactions.

The more mature depression can be suspended to foster regression to the less mature reaction. Psychological reflective techniques are highly applicable to the more mature depression. However, if this more mature reaction is mistaken for an anaclitic reaction, the risk of further internalization of rage and irritation is present. Comfort and solace are usually contraindicated for more mature depressive reactions. They foster internalization rather than permit a venting of anger within the analysis. The result is continued self-containment, which is carcinogenic in that it serves as an irritant.

The anaclitic stage of depression can also be diagnosed when a relatively sudden shift occurs within the therapeutic relationship. With more mature defenses, the patient's inability to express certain problems within the therapeutic relationship may be viewed as a "transference resistance." It is anticipation of the analyst's reaction to what could be said that inhibits the expression of feelings.

Most people are not raised in an emotional environment that permits them to express all feelings freely. Children are taught that certain things are not permissible in an exchange with parents. The more primitive the feeling, the closer the feeling brings the child to hate or sex, the more inhibitions are placed upon the communication of them. This occurs within the initial emotional training as well as in the surrogate relationship of analysis. A major aspect of the analyst's task is to suspend the defenses that surround the expression of sexual or murderous feelings within the analysis. These are part of the constellation of defenses that compose the repetition compulsion, that is, the need to repeat that in which we are emotionally invested and with which we are familiar. Once the analytic relationship forms, defenses against the expression of forbidden feelings, with the analyst as the object, are termed *transference resistances*. Transference resistances are a frequent occurrence in the course of any analysis.

There is another form of defense related to this surrogate maternal relationship, which is called "resistance to transference." It usually is encountered first in a therapeutic relationship with a patient who appears disconnected and out of touch with his surroundings. It is as if the patient does not want any relationship to develop and, yet, paradoxically, maintains his appointments and follows the analytic rules in general.

The analyst will need to guard against feelings of not being interested in such an individual. He may be bored, sleepy, or annoyed during sessions. It may appear to him that the patient could just as well be talking to a tape recorder as another human being. If the patient asks questions, they are either rhetorical or the patient will answer them himself, frequently just as the analyst is about to respond. To deal with this apparently pointless situation, the analyst may investigate the patterns of defense by asking the patient why he does not ask real questions. He may also ask the patient how he perceives him. The purpose of such gentle questioning is to grant permission subtly to the patient to relate to the surrogate mother.

Other patients may appear confident and highly verbal. They will describe life events as if the sun rises and sets only upon them. But all of their narcissistic egocentric defenses are compensations. They cover the insecurities and self-hate of the person too frightened to relate to others. Fragility will be sensed by the experienced sensitive analyst. *The fear of relating is what is dominant.*

In dealing with the precancerous and many cancerous individuals, treatment may progress through very understandable elements of transference resistance. One of the most significant symptoms of regression to an anaclitic depression will be a shift in feelings within the relationship. From perhaps moderate feelings of hatred and love, the patient seems suddenly to stop the process. It may seem as if the treatment was just beginning with regard to building a relationship when an apparent resistance to transference (resistance to relating) suddenly develops.

The patient may use adult rationalizations like "I've outgrown you" or "You're just another person like every one else." The analyst may actually feel hurt by this lack of involvement after, perhaps, a long time of dealing with moderated feelings, but he should stop and examine thoroughly the process of treatment up to this point. *Did he provoke such a reaction within his patient by not allowing the emergence of primitive feelings?* If he can find no evidence of this counterdefense, then he should suspect the evolution of the anaclitic depression within the analytic relationship. It will appear to be a sudden shift from "transference resistance" to "resistance to transference." In other words, it will appear to be a shift from fear of expressing feelings that obviously exist to a fear of relating at all.

This marks the beginning of the regression to the infantile depression that serves as a final line of defense against the primitive feelings of raw irritation and homeostasis. This shift marks the point in treatment at which the analyst must stop using psychological reflective techniques. The rage of the anaclitic depression is used to defend against the impending annihilation of the negative autistic stage. Once the pushing away stops, the objections to impingements stop, and the expression of rage and then irritation must be welcomed and accepted by the analyst. The integrating of the expression of autistic-stage homeostasis and irritation can be experienced by the analyst as one of the genuine rewards of his work. No one will thank him for it, certainly not the precancer or cancer patients he treats. But the analyst can now enjoy the increased probability of the survival of his patient. As he meets raw irritation with acceptance and caring, he conditions a fusion. He is also conditioning a new mechanism to deal with all irritation.

The genetic damage to precancer or cancer patients seems unlikely to be reversed once a genetic translocation has taken place. What the analyst is accomplishing is a reconditioning of the handling of irritation. From inner directed, the patient becomes outer directed. From hypersensitive, the patient becomes capable of modulating feelings. Events that would have had his endocrine system on overtime are now accepted as the foibles of life.

The analyst has provided a mechanism to lessen the impact of the internalized irritations of the autistic stage. Love has been demonstrated to heighten the efficiency of the immunological system.

Physicians and laymen alike are aware of the importance of psychological states in susceptibility and resistance to disease. To a certain extent, people can learn to deal with stress and anxiety on their own. However, for a reversal of the cancerous process to occur, another human being must play a part in the recovery of health. It is not easy to convince the cancer patient of this. The beginning stages of psychoanalytic treatment of the cancer patient will frequently be marked by a defense against relating to others that may come much later for a precancer patient. In both cases, however, this is a defense against immediate annihilation at the autistic level. There is a genuine fear of coming into contact with primitive feelings. The patient's expectation because of his original conditioning is that his irritations will be met by overwhelming irritation.

Therefore, although analysis is obviously the least toxic approach to cancer when compared to chemotherapy, radiology, or surgery, with the fewest side effects and minimal risk, the reaction of the patient to the analyst can seem hard to understand. From direct accusations of charlantanism to stating quietly "It's just not for me," a concerned friend or relative may be surprised at the patient's not only lacking desire for, but obstinately avoiding, the analytic process. A typical conversation might go something like this:

Relative: What did you think of your first visit?
Patient: I thought she was a nice lady, but it's not for me.
Relative: Why not?
Patient: It's just not for me. Analysis is for crazy people. I'm not crazy. I have cancer. She can't help. It's not for me.
Relative: She sees a lot of people who aren't crazy, and she helps them a lot in their lives. Why not give it a try?
Patient: Look, I really appreciate your concern, but I'm not a candidate for that. It's too late for me anyway. You know that.

Arguing with the patient is usually to no avail because of the patient's unconscious need to repeat the anaclitic depressive position. The fear of dealing with the feelings that this infantile depression guards against is equivalent to a fear of immediate annihilation.

How then can someone with cancer be motivated to face his fears of emotional death prior to a real physical death? The physician can help. The patient already trusts him to carry out all sorts of potentially hazardous procedures. If he genuinely believes that cancer may have a significant emotional basis, the cancer specialist will be able to demonstrate her caring by making such a referral. The patient, like the infant, will sense the unspoken feelings.

Another way to motivate the cancer patient to seek out a competent psychoanalyst is to have him read this book. A cancer patient will see himself in these pages. The adult, logical part of his mind might just be able to use all of this information to face his fears of the feelings behind the infantile depression.

In summary, the psychoanalytic treatment plan for a pre-cancer or cancer patient is direct and simple to understand. First, a suspension of more advanced defenses must take place so that the anaclitic depressive position is reached. If cancer already exists, it will assist in facilitating this regression. As the individual is overwhelmed by his fears, the more advanced stages of defense will no longer work effectively. In order to get past these more advanced stages of defense, an implementation of reflective techniques is strongly recommended. Avoid using interpretation or insight therapies. Avoid artificial gestaltlike conjuring of images. Instead, work to build an early surrogate maternal relationship.

The second stage may take quite some time, as in the case of a precancerous condition, or it may be reached quickly, as in the case of an active cancer. Once the regression reaches the anaclitic depression, the patient will desperately push away from the analyst. Destruction of treatment is a very great risk. If the analyst ignores, or is unaware of, the fact that the patient is trying to avoid the feelings behind the cancer, the patient will have to flee. If the analyst ignores the fact that he, the analyst, represents the cancer in the patient's unconscious, then the patient will have to flee. And if the analyst continues psychological reflection after the patient has reached autism, the cancer will worsen. If the analyst can first be viewed as the ultimate carcinogen, irritant, or cancer itself, and if he then can offer love and caring when the patient wants to flee from or destroy the analyst, a reconditioning can occur. A fusion of basic psychological forces will ensue as the patient learns to dissipate irritation through emotional entropy.

13

Karen

Und wie dein Wille ihren Sinn begreift,
lassen sie deine Augen zartlich los.

(From Eingang [Initiation] by R. M. Rilke)

When you have grasped its meaning with your will,
then tenderly your eyes will let it go.
(Translated by C. F. MacIntyre in *Rilke, Selected Poems*)

FOR ME SHE WAS WHERE THIS all began, over a dozen years ago. At the time we met, all of the trite descriptions of a person wasting away fit her. Her skin was pale gray, with a clammy look to it. The dark semicircles under her eyes made her appear exhausted and terribly depressed. Her eyes bulged from her face and appeared glazed, dull, almost lifeless. She stared off into space, lost in her solitude. It did not take me long to realize that when she looked at me, she was seeing nothing.

Chemotherapy had caused most of Karen's hair to fall out. But the most shocking aspect of her appearance was her emaciation. She looked as if she had very recently been liberated from

Auschwitz. Her skin clung to her skeleton. Her cheeks were concave. Both feet seemed to be already in the grave. All that remained was for her to lie down and be still.

When she first entered my office, she needed her husband's and mother's moral and physical support. She could barely walk.

Two days earlier, I had received a call from Dr. G., who works at one of the most famous cancer centers on the East Coast. He asked if I had had any success with treating drug abusers. Of course I answered yes. I was the clinical director of a drug abuse agency.

He asked me if I would help a patient of his cut down on pain medication. He explained that Karen was a twenty-six-year-old cancer patient who had had all the possible medical treatment, with no beneficial results. She had had a colostomy, but another malignant tumor had developed ten months later. She had had radiation and chemotherapy to the limit. And she had begun using Percodan more for emotional problems than for pain, so that when the time came that she would really need it, it wouldn't have any effect.

I asked Dr. G. for her prognosis, and he replied with one word: "Hopeless." When I asked about how much time she had to live, Dr. G. assured me that Karen had at the most three to six months, but he believed it more reasonable to anticipate her death within the next three months.

At this point, for some reason, I restrained myself. I didn't want to tell Dr. G. that I had never "cured" anyone of drug abuse within a few weeks of the beginning of treatment. And I did not want to ask him the ultimate question: why bother if she had only a relatively rapid and certain death to look forward to. Most of all, I did not want to say no, I won't, or can't, do it. I still do not know why I didn't want to.

Karen's mother and husband left the office after they had helped seat her comfortably. She asked me what she should talk about. I told her that she could tell me everything and that her job was just to talk.

What did I mean by everything, she wanted to know. I explained that she should say anything that she wanted to say. She could tell me the story of her life if she wished. For the next ten minutes, she talked about how depressed she was over having to leave her children. Her children were six and three and a half years old. The older was a boy, the younger a girl.

Death was, thus, first portrayed by Karen as a separation. She described her cancer in a cool clinical manner, talking of her pain and discomfort as if she were speaking of someone else. But when it came to her two small children being left without her, her voice quaked, and she fought back the tears. In adult language, she spoke for them, for their inability to understand, and for their sadness and anger over her leaving them.

I felt like crying at several points but worked to control myself and to remain relatively quiet. I asked three or four neutral questions to distract her from the powerful feelings she was expressing. My fear was that she would reveal too much too soon and then be too embarrassed to continue the treatment.

By the time the first session was over, we had agreed to meet twice a week. She seemed slightly more energetic at the conclusion of the session. She extended her hand, and I shook it. Then, I asked her what the handshake meant in words. "Thanks" was all she said and left.

I was completely exhausted emotionally. On very few occasions have I felt so depressed. I knew that *I* could not handle this alone. I had just begun my training at a psychoanalytic institute where Mrs. Yonata Feldman was on the faculty, and I decided to ask her to be my case supervisor. Perhaps her forty years of experience could make up for my near-total deficiency in this regard. Fortunately, she agreed. Supervision was on a group level, and Karen's case was picked to be presented each week.

After my first presentation of the little I knew about Karen, Mrs. Feldman sat quietly listening to the irrelevant questions and comments of this group of novices. When they finally finished, she tilted slightly forward and asked, "Can he do it?" Her usual grandmotherly benevolent smile was gone. She sat impassively, her mouth a straight line bridging her round cheeks, emphasizing her seriousness.

The first student to speak, a middle-aged man with the classical look of an analyst—goatee, glasses, and elbow-patched Harristweed jacket—said he felt Mrs. Feldman was asking if I could cure my young patient of cancer. He also said that if this was the meaning of her question, then she was being cruel and unfair to me. After all, the physician had said that Karen would certainly be dead within six months at the most.

Mrs. Feldman's only comment on this point was that his interpretation of the original question was correct. She was asking if I could *cure* the cancer. One by one, the students, all seven of them, agreed it was hopeless. A doctor with a central European accent offered me an out. "Perhaps," she said, "a cure could have been possible, but this cancer is obviously too far advanced."

Mrs. Feldman looked down at the desktop, remaining silent for what seemed like hours but was only moments. She was reflecting upon something. I was studying her hands. At first they were tightly clasped together. Suddenly, she leaned even farther forward, unclasped her hands, placed them squarely on the desk, and stared into my eyes. I returned the stare and saw a certain impish sparkle in her eyes. "Can you do it, young man?" she asked. "Can you cure this woman's cancer?" Her eyes continued to look into mine. For a moment, I could not talk. I wanted to say yes, unequivocally, but I did not feel it. I knew that was what she wanted, but the best I could offer was an inane, nondescript "maybe."

She looked down at her hands. The gleam left her eyes. I felt as though I had deeply wounded her, violated her. I regrouped my forces. "Yes, I can, with your help. I can do it."

Mrs. Feldman's mouth turned up into a huge contagious smile. That is, it was contagious for me—no one else in the class smiled. They didn't understand that I needed hope. They didn't understand that my patient needed hope. They didn't understand that Yonata Feldman knew there was always hope if life and feeling were within reach. At that point, I loved her for the gift that was to take thirteen years to cultivate and mature. When Yonata Feldman died recently, I suffered a great loss. So did you.

The next session with Karen brought more surprises. She entered my office smartly attired, wearing a high-fashion wig and makeup. This was quite a shock for me. Obviously, no matter how meticulously a "terminal" cancer patient attends to her grooming, her appearance still reflects the effect of cancer and cachexia. So, there was something almost Felliniesque about the way Karen looked. Her denial of death seemed almost absurd.

The real absurdity, however, was my denial. It took Mrs. Feldman by surprise that I did not recognize Karen's behavior as an attempt at *seduction.* For months the patient had let her appearance deteriorate. All of a sudden, she was working desperately at looking as good as she possibly could, and all I saw was that the rouge on her sunken gray cheeks made her look like a sickly pathetic clown.

When Mrs. Feldman used the word seduction in explaining this to me, I felt like the proverbial Missouri mule. First, you have to get his attention; then, he can learn anything. The best attention getter for a Missouri mule is a two-by-four between the ears. This tunes him in. When Mrs. Feldman used the word seduction, I felt as if I had been hit with a two-by-four.

At this point in my training analysis and education, I did not recognize that I was resistant to seeing this obvious communication for what it was. I was nowhere near ready to know that fusion with Karen would be necessary for her cure. I was nowhere near ready to recognize that being relatively unanalyzed myself was putting me in any kind of danger of cancer. However, it took only this one smack with the two-by-four to open my eyes.

The courtship continued until the end of Karen's treatment. Let me hasten to add that behavior suggesting courting never took place. The thoughts and, more important, the feelings were sufficient. Karen was a very proper, very Catholic, parochial school graduate. She had also attended a Catholic women's college. Acting out was never even a remote risk to the treatment. No statements of wanting such intimacy were ever directly or consciously made. When she had dreams of a fusional relationship with her analyst, the fusion always precluded genital sexuality. In the dream I would be holding her, walking someplace with her, touching her face; or I would be a swarm of vicious insects invading her body and devouring her from the inside out. The fusion was there, but it was extreme in terms of hyperirritation or homeostasis. I was either the mother who cared for her feelings through emotional entropy, or I was the mother who added irritation to preexisting irritation. I was the mother who comforted and soothed, or I was her cancer. I knew nothing of this at the time.

When Karen asked if we could go for a walk one fine spring afternoon, I was very much tempted. But I realized that to do so I would have to support her physically and used this as my rationalization for not going along with her wish. Instead I told her how great I felt that she wanted to do this with me. I talked about where we should walk, whether we could rest along the way, and what she might want to share seeing with me.

When Karen told me she wanted to see the buds on the trees and show me her favorite Japanese maple, my eyes misted over. Could Yonata Feldman have been right? When I reported Karen's wish in class, Mrs. Feldman's eyes seemed to fill with tears. I don't think this was my projection; I think the tears were real.

Half-jokingly Karen had said, "Springtime and death just simply don't go together." I asked her what does go well with springtime, and she answered, "Babies, flowers, lovers, and mostly romance, but not in that order."

She described her husband's courtship and how wonderful he had been. She repeatedly emphasized what a wonderful man he was, so sensitive and vulnerable. She described him as playful, almost mischievous, at times. But as she continued her description of him and the marital relationship, it became clear that she was consistently in the maternal role, soothing and comforting him. She was completely unaware of how little her husband was giving her emotionally. She saw her task in life as that of caring for the needs of others. This obviously included her two children, but what was not so obvious was her third baby: her husband.

Adding to the problem was the fact that Hal, her husband, was a Protestant. Karen's parents had almost totally disowned her at the time of her marriage, and when she refused to have her children baptized, all communication stopped. She was an abandoned child, and she remained an abandoned child until she was diagnosed as having cancer. She still would not have contacted her parents, but Hal called them. In the face of such horror, they suspended the rejection of their daughter. They felt guilty, and they admitted this to Karen. She, on the other hand, hated them for what had transpired. On some level, she realized that they had treated her as if she were a leper—or as if she had died. Was she then living up to the role they had prescribed?

Karen described her mother as cold and unaffectionate. As a child, she could recall the peck on the cheek kisses, the lack of hugs, and the almost nonexistent verbal communication. Every Christmas, the perfect gift was left under the tree, but never with a meaningful card. "Mom considered that stuff corny," she said. "It was simply 'To Karen, from Mom.'" More often, there was no "to" or "from" on any emotional level. While Karen obviously could not recall her early infancy, it was a safe bet that her mother was intermittently emotionally unresponsive. She behaved properly more out of guilt or concern for doing the right thing than out of love and caring.

In the course of her treatment, I had the opportunity to meet with her family members. Karen's mother lived up to her daughter's description. She was bright, affable, extremely proper, and egocentric. She kept referring to the fact that her daughter's death was a certainty but that she, the mother, could not accept it. She spoke of the burden of caring for her dying daughter. And she spoke of the future burden of caring for her grandchildren. At least, she did recognize that her son-in-law could not possibly cope.

In the few sessions I had with her, she never once referred to her daughter's feelings or pain except in terms of their effect on herself. For example, she would say, "I really can't deal with Karen's suffering. It makes *me* feel sick to have to see a child of mine suffer so."

After several weeks, Karen's coloring changed. The grayish, clammy hue was replaced by a paleness that many fair-skinned redheads or blondes have. I called Dr. G. to tell him about it, and he asked whether she was reporting any change in appetite and eating habits. At the next session, I asked Karen about this.

She replied, "I guess I have been eating a little more. Come to think of it I am eating maybe six or seven little meals each day. And you know what? I am not throwing it up like when I was on chemo or afterward. You know I didn't even realize this was happening. How did you know to ask me that?"

I told her that she was looking much better to me. Strangely this compliment seemed almost to startle her. She immediately began to describe her never-ending pain. She sounded almost defensive and somewhat angry. Apparently she was not ready to give up any of her symptoms consciously. I had inadvertently attacked her defenses with my very mild compliment.

After the shock wore off, I told her that she looked better only because of her new skin color. I quickly added that it might not mean anything. Again, I was surprised by her reaction, this time to my pessimism. She blushed and looked down in an almost coquettish manner. To put it as succinctly as possible: *I was totally confused!* When I complimented her, she felt attacked, and when I told her she was probably not getting better, she became a little girl flirting with me!

Mrs. Feldman explained that I was reflecting the defense (resistance) when I expressed pessimism. That freed the feelings beneath the surface. The blush came from Karen's feeling understood and then getting in touch with her desire for caring and loving.

But it may have been too soon. It may have been an intuitive joining on my part, but the premature release of such powerful feelings could destroy the treatment. The feelings could scare the little baby Karen was concealing within her, and she might have to flee or be overwhelmed.

Mrs. Feldman told me to limit myself to two to five neutral questions per session. She warned me against making statements of any kind, particularly any that could so easily be misconstrued as a compliment. Any need to gratify my or Dr. G.'s curiosity would have to be controlled. It was not in Karen's best interest, and it was potentially far too risky.

After several months of treatment, she began to gain weight for the first time in over a year, and she continued to gain weight as she passed the six-month survival limit of Dr. G.'s prognosis. She actually appeared to be getting better. Remission, an unexplainable remission, is what the doctors called it.

Yonata Feldman pointed out to me that the defense of self-destruction was no longer operating. In hindsight I would say that the conditioned response of cancer had been extinguished. But why? No one had an adequate explanation. Mrs. Feldman's interpretation only told me what was obvious. Karen, however, was telling me through her dreams and fantasies. All I had to do was hear her words. Her unconscious was rich in vivid imagery that portrayed her struggle against her totally regressive death.

It was the winter of the first year of her new life. She walked into my office under her own steam, looking vibrant and alive.

Her eyes had a twinkle in them, and she looked as if she could be modeling for *Vogue*. Her hair was growing back, and she wore it in a stylish short cut. She was dressed in a lacy white blouse with a black skirt and patterned stockings. For the first time, I was able to see how attractive she really was.

Karen: I went to a PTA meeting. Can you believe that? I actually felt good enough to get out of the house and go. Some people I know just as acquaintances did not recognize me. A few who did complimented me on my weight loss and new hair style. They said I looked great. I told them to just keep talking and not to stop. (Pause) What do you think?

Analyst: Would that matter?

Karen: Yes it would, or I wouldn't ask.

Analyst: What if I thought you looked horrendous? [I was trying to follow what I thought was my analytic role.]

Karen: I'd be crushed. But just answer me. Cut the questions and answer me!

Analyst: You look wonderful. [I was afraid to continue frustrating her, and I was also afraid to be so complimentary. I hoped my supervisor could help me pick up the pieces in the aftermath of the compliment.]

Karen: You answered! Do you really think I look good?

Analyst: No, I think you're a pretty ugly person. I always tell ugly people they look great. It's one of my eccentricities.

Karen: You are a character. But you're right. I should know if I look good. I just wanted to hear it from you.

Analyst: What makes my opinion important?

Karen: Oh, cut it out! You know I care what you think about everything. [A repetition of the early maternal relationship.] You're very important to me. Maybe, sometimes, I think you are too important. But enough of that. Let me tell you a weird dream I had.

216

It started off with Hal and me going on a vacation to Florida. He's a nut about fishing, and when we're there, he goes out on a boat every day. I stay on some quiet beach and read a novel. Anyway, in the dream I went out in this little boat with him. The water was beautiful. The colors were all in pastel blues and greens. Islands dotted the stillness of the flats, as Hal calls this fishing area. I was in a bikini, baking in the sun. He was wearing cutoffs and a silly fishing hat as he was casting from the front of the boat. It was all very sensual.

Two dolphins suddenly appeared next to the boat. At first, I thought they were sharks because of the dorsal fins, but then they stuck their faces out of the water and chattered away at us. I threw them some bait fish, and they squealed with delight. Then, suddenly, they turned and swam away to join other dolphins off in the distance. They were gone. Maybe they represent the kids. I don't know.

But anyway, Hal hooked into a big fish. His rod was almost bent in half when he flipped it into the boat. It almost landed on me. It was silvery, with a big mouth. But when it hit the deck right next to me, it sort of shattered into pieces. The pieces became little silvery fish with ugly mouths and sharp teeth. They went for me. I saw them going for my stomach. They were like vermin attached to me with needlelike teeth. If I tried to pull them off, I tore my flesh. I was bleeding.

Out of nowhere, this handsome muscular guy appeared. He grabbed each fish and crushed it as it hung on me. After he killed them, he opened their mouths by pressing on the sides of the jaws. The teeth came out of me. He threw them back in the water. But they turned back into the big silver fish that Hal had caught. I looked up to see this guy's face, but the sun blinded me

217

so that I had to look away. He put some kind of lotion or medicine on each wound. His hands and arms looked powerful and rough, but his touch was gentle, even tender. No one said a word.

He climbed onto a platform at the back of the boat. In real life, guides usually do this and push the boats along with a long pole from back there. He was doing that. I realized that Hal had just disappeared from the scene. Again I tried to see this guy's face, and again the sun was in my eyes. I looked down at his feet and worked my way up his legs; they were gorgeous. Tanned skin with powerful muscles. Veins showed through, and normally that turns me off, but not this time. The hair on his legs was blondish. I kept looking up, but as soon as I saw *his* tight-fitting cutoffs, I woke up.

I tried to get back to sleep in order to continue the dream, but I couldn't, or if I did, I don't remember it. I guess I woke up because I was getting to forbidden feelings about someone other than my husband. I also was upset when I thought that all the dead little fish turned back into that big one, and it just swam away. I had the thought that it swam away to be caught another day. I don't know why, but that made me feel empty inside.

When I told Mrs. Feldman about this, she emphasized that Karen was getting in touch with issues of closeness in the treatment. She said that this was the critical issue. She must not be allowed to use sexuality as an excuse to avoid real maternal closeness. I was advised to avoid any questioning or comments that even tangentially could bring us to the issue of adult sexuality.

Karen's symbols for cancer and her detached relationship with her husband were connected in the fish her husband caught and the predatory little fish that began to consume her. All the Freudian symbols of waving a "rod" around were joked about by the class until Mrs. Feldman pointed out that Hal's lack of involvement with his wife might be related to her cancer.

The guide was generally viewed as a representative of me, the analyst. One woman jokingly asked how I looked in cutoffs. I told her I had knobby knees.

The blinding sun was seen as Karen's defense against being consciously aware of sexual feelings toward me. Everyone in the class, myself included, related this to her strict religious upbringing and a desire for treatment to continue. If she had realized that her "guide" represented her analyst, she might have had to destroy treatment out of false guilt at being unfaithful in her marriage. Unfortunately, Karen believed that a thought was equivalent to a deed.

Looking back over the years at this dream, I became aware of the screen that the macho guide provided to prevent Karen from knowing that she desired a maternal fusion and emotional entropy. Sex was a superficial issue. This "guide" saved her life and then continued to steer the course. Had she been able to see his face and desire his body, things might have been very different.

I believe now that these matters should have been explored. In some way, Karen should have been made to understand that *feelings* of adultery do not get anyone into divorce court. The big fish that got away to be caught another day might *not* have if her feelings had been dealt with as they evolved. The potential destruction of the treatment came from not teaching her how to tolerate such emotions.

This dream demonstrates that cancer patients do not have to conjure up images of their disorder or their protectors artifically. They do it quite spontaneously, naturally.

After the second year of Karen's treatment, an unanticipated question arose in class. How come the treatment was continuing?

Dr. G. had only asked for assistance in lowering her drug intake; that had been accomplished within several months of the start of her therapy. Now she was totally drug free.

She had never raised the question of not continuing, and it had never occurred to me. Obviously a relationship had developed in which drugs or even cancer were secondary to feelings of connection. The process of her treatment seemed so natural that no one had questioned it until this point.

Added to this was the fact that by now Karen had no sign of cancer anywhere in her body. It just seemed to have happened. Some of the medical people said that, perhaps, all the techniques they had utilized were finally working. Dr. G. said he had no explanation. He had seen people outlive their prognosis, but Karen was more than just holding on. He had heard of spontaneous cures, but he had witnessed none previously in his career. He jokingly said that I should "bottle" whatever I was doing with Karen.

But I still had a very limited knowledge of what I actually was doing. Mrs. Feldman, however, was enjoying every minute of the case presentation. She, at least, seemed to know something the rest of us were in the dark about.

Karen continued to tell me the story of her life and, eventually, began to see that Hal was inadequate at meeting her emotional needs. She described him as basically immature and more interested in his friends than his wife. She had always been impressed with his ability to play with the children until she became aware that he was playing as a peer, not a father. He even had trouble letting the children win at games. She complained that although they had resumed their sex life, nothing had really changed. Gratification was frequently unilateral, and afterward there was no holding, talking, or tenderness. He just went to sleep.

For weeks prior to the return of their sexual relations, Karen had expressed her fear of being repulsive to Hal because of the scars left by surgery and radiation. She was afraid that he would not be able to be aroused by someone so disfigured, but the real crushing blow came when she realized that he did not even seem to notice.

At first, she thought he was just protecting her feelings by saying nothing and appearing oblivious. However, when she commented on it to him, he sort of shrugged and said it was "no big deal."

To Karen this was an intolerable negation of her feelings. "Why couldn't he have said he loved me so much that it was no big deal?" she asked. "Or maybe that I was such a turn-on, it was no big deal. The way he said it, it sounded like my feelings and fears of rejection were unimportant. I was genuinely shocked by the way he reacted. I don't know if I can ever forgive him for that!"

Karen continued to complain about Hal's insensitivity. She came to realize that he was, in many ways, far more like her mother than her father. The more she complained about him, the more interested she became in me. Why wasn't I wearing a wedding ring? How old was I anyway? Where did I go to school? The questions were a part of almost every session. I explored all of them with her rather than answering directly. When she asked about my age, for example, rather than simply answer, the matter was explored.

When she asked about my marital status, she told me that because she preferred to think of me as single, I would be single in her mind. This conversation evolved into what type of woman I would be interested in. She speculated that my choice would be bright, well-educated, and voluptuous in appearance. Interestingly this was a good description of Karen, even though she did not see herself as such. Karen was thinking of my hypothetical ideal female as someone other than herself. This may have been an attempt at creating distance and denying her feelings.

As she denigrated her husband and became more and more interested in her analyst, the little girl coquettishness disappeared. She began to share the intimacies of her *secret* past: episodes of cheating in school, experimenting with drugs and sex. She was a child of the sixties and had been caught between the religious influences on her and the liberated atmosphere that surrounded her generation. Hesitantly she revealed that she and Hal had participated in peace demonstrations even though her priest and parents supported the war in Vietnam. This placed her in still another conflict for she admitted that her peace activities were as much for socializing and fun as for any real convictions about the war. She now condemned herself for lack of purity of purpose.

A sense of propriety permeated her existence. When things were not right in her small world, or the world at large as she saw it, it genuinely irritated her. From the minute to the enormous, everything had its place or an upset resulted. The apparent lack of reason behind, as well as the lack of cause for, the Vietnam war made it a tremendous irritant to Karen. When she had permitted herself to belong, to feel part of, that is, enjoy, the peace movement, she had been brought in touch with the intimacy of fusion. Her guilt about not taking it seriously enough can thus be viewed as an attempt at diluting the feelings of belonging.

As she became aware that even subtle seduction would not work, she became less interested in me. The less interested she appeared to be in me as a significant entity in her life, the more she revealed about her most intimate thoughts and feelings. But when I could be trusted with such important aspects of her life, I was placed in what seemed like a less important and less intense role. At least, it appeared to me, that I was less significant emotionally. And as I became less significant emotionally, Karen became more and more depressed. I did not know it at the time, but I believe now that this strange paradox indicated that she was entering an anaclitic depression.

She began to speak in philosophical existential terms about the meaning of life. Love and hate were discussed as vague uncertain feelings. Karen attacked herself for doubting her love for her husband, even her children at times. She admitted not knowing what love was. Although she had all the acceptable responses, she felt that they were shallow and empty. She cried when she said she might never have really experienced such closeness. Her inadequate mother, once again, became a topic; and then, for the first time, Karen tied her husband to her mother.

I asked where *I* fit in. She said she did not know; however, I was slipping away. Karen seemed saddened when she said she did not understand why, but that I was not nearly as significant a part of her life as I had been.

Instead of recognizing this shift to the anaclitic depression, I felt rejected and hurt. Mrs. Feldman and, now, even the class seemed to think that I was probably responsible for her recovery. Even if I did not really believe that I had done anything to help, I certainly wanted to. This made Karen's confusion an attack upon me. I was narcissistically wounded. I cared more about my feelings than hers. In my mind she became an ingrate.

What I did not realize was that she was becoming a small baby whose fears centered upon closeness, a closeness that meant annihilation. She had to reduce the intimacy in order to avoid the annihilation she was taught to fear. At one point, she told me I was talking too much. I looked back on the session and realized I had said almost nothing, but the little I did say was perceived as an enormous irritation. Karen reacted to whatever I said as if my voice grated upon her. Instead of recognizing the hypersensitive baby, I saw an adult woman showing me I was unsatisfactory. In my ignorance, I was vulnerable. In hindsight it is all too clear what had happened. My lack of understanding helped lead to the inevitable premature end of Karen's treatment.

At this point in my training and Karen's analysis, we both suffered a tremendous loss. Mrs. Feldman's health was deteriorating, and she was in and out of hospitals. Her mysticism and twinkle were no longer there for us. She had had a way of getting all of us to do the right things with our patients. No one else has had such a powerful effect upon my education. Yonata Feldman's internal little girl was insistent upon not being disappointed or denied. At the same time, she was totally supportive in the way she made recommendations. Now she was unavailable. I felt like a little boy cast out into a tough world long before I was ready. I was angry with Mrs. Feldman for getting sick, but I pushed this out of my mind and instead clung to superficial realities. I would have to make do with someone else.

I am sure that the loss of Mrs. Feldman as my supervisor was far more important than the competence of the man who took her place. I had felt that I was in over my head right from my first session with Karen, but Mrs. Feldman had repeatedly thrown me a life preserver. I listened to my highly competent new supervisor, but I did not hear him.

Karen continued to demean our relationship. She told me that I was becoming real, that my magic was leaving. "You are like everyone else," she said. "I see you as smart but not all knowing. Cute maybe, but you'd never be a movie star. Something is gone. I feel the loss, but I'm afraid it will never be back."

My new supervisor told me to give her space and, in effect, allow the dilution. This made sense if the best treatment plan was to continue to be nonconfrontative. What neither one of us saw was the suicide lurking behind Karen's pushing away. Like the foundling-home baby, she should not have been put down. I put her down. I allowed her to push away. I did not take advantage of the fact that she was at this point still ambivalent.

Karen: I don't know why we are continuing. The last test series at the hospital showed that no active cancer exists anywhere in my body. So why are we continuing? I'm not taking any medication either.

Analyst: Maybe we should consider stopping.

Karen: When you say that my body feels weird. I sort of float
           from my stomach, and I tingle all over. My arms and
           legs are heavy and light at the same time. I don't think I
           could walk if I had to. All this happened as soon as you
           said maybe we should stop. I'd be too scared to stop.
           Leaving you frightens me. But I hate being so depend-
           ent!

I received all sorts of advice from my new supervisor. None of it
made sense or seemed applicable. I, too, was a baby who had been
put down. I felt toward my new supervisor what Karen felt
toward me. We were getting nowhere, but I was afraid to leave
him. Then it happened.

Karen had another dream. This was the last dream Karen ever
told me about. It sealed the fate of her treatment and thus,
indirectly, her entire fate. She used this dream to destroy our
relationship, and I (and my supervisor) did not know how to stop
it. We also did not know what the horrible consequences would
be.

Karen: I had a very upsetting dream last night. It made me feel
           horrible, even though I knew it was entirely absurd.
Analyst: The more absurd, the better.
Karen: I was being chased by a huge red lobster. The claws
           kept snapping shut with the loudness of a gunshot. All
           of a sudden, Hal appeared and was holding my hand,
           and we both ran as fast as we could. I got the feeling
           that he was slowing me down, that I could get caught in
           the lobster's claws. The scene ends, and just as sud-
           denly, I'm in a new scene.

           I am with you and Hal. The lobster is gone, and we
           are just walking somewhere. You are on my right, and
           Hal is on my left. Hal disappears, and it is just you and

me. We stop and hug. That's when I woke up. As soon as I woke up, I thought that the dream meant I want you and not Hal. Hal is the father of my children. He has seen me through all sorts of difficulties. It's absurd that I would reject him for anyone.

Of course I pointed out that this was only a dream. I told her that dreams don't simply mean what the surface story tells. And I asked her why having the feelings was so objectionable when there were no actions. She nervously dismissed everything I said as analytic poppycock. At the same time, she said she was confused and could not understand what I said.

The worst happened. She was unconsciously recognizing her marriage's contribution to her cancer (the lobster). And she was recognizing the powerful need to replace those dynamics with something better. The trouble was that she still equated the feeling with the deed. The thought of ending her marriage was overwhelmingly frightening to her.

Karen started missing sessions. Several weeks later, she decided to end her analysis. I offered all sorts of good reasons to continue. She seemed to agree with all of them and then dismissed them as meaningless. Two years and ten months after we first met, Karen's treatment ended. As far as the medical experts were concerned, there was no sign of active cancer in her body. Three years and three months after our first meeting, Karen was dead from cancer.

Within one month after treatment stopped, Karen was diagnosed as having widespread cancer, similar to, but even more pervasive than, what she had when her analysis began. Four months later she died. I was devastated when Hal called and told me what had happened.

Dr. G. told me that it was a very unusual reoccurrence, unusual in the degree of spreading and the rapidity of tumor growth.

He said that the cancer must have been just below the surface for the entire time.

I believe that Karen died because I mistakenly put the baby down.

Karen provided the impetus for the evolution of my theory of the causes and prevention of cancer. My ultimate failure in treating her was based upon my ignorance. The strangeness of her death helped open my eyes. I hope it has opened the readers' as well.

But most important, I hope that some of the mystery of cancer is now at least a little less mysterious. Perhaps the reader can now view the supposed inevitability of the disorder as within his or her power to influence significantly.

14

Conclusions

I COULD HAVE WAITED. THE ghost of the ancient Greek physician Galen is still waiting. It was in 537 B.C.—that's right, 537 B.C.—that he noticed that internalizing, melancholy women were more prone to breast cancer than outgoing, cheerful women. In 1926, Dr. Elida Evans studied one hundred cancer patients and found that the loss of a significant relationship was the most common predisposing factor. Out of five hundred cancer patients recently studied by Dr. L. LeShan, 72 percent demonstrated the following pattern:

1. A childhood marked by depression and isolation.

2. Poor parental relationships.

3. A return to feelings similar to the isolation and despair of their childhoods.

4. Loss of a job or relationship that had strong emotions attached. Within six to eight months after the loss, cancer appeared.

Only 10 percent of the noncancer control group had this history.

Doctors Evans and LeShan are still waiting for a theory that integrates their observations with the facts of carcinogen theory, virology, nutrition, and dynamic psychology. I believe my theory

229

succeeds at this integration. It fills in the blanks and appears to be able to address all the aspects of cancer.

The logic behind it provides answers to why certain areas of our bodies are relatively immune to cancer. It provides answers to the mysteries of spontaneous cures. It explains the phenomenon intrinsic to medical treatment. It provides an orientation for prevention and cure. At this point, we have observable fact coupled with theoretical causation. If we integrate the use of oncological medical techniques with the patient's psychology, we will maximize the effectiveness of these techniques. If we stop worshipping minutia, we will be able to see the entire patient in his life space. If we do not, we will continue to spend millions on useless studies that only demonstrate the obvious.

But some readers of this book will still wait. Wait for what, you might ask. Wait for more proof—some people will demand that I cure a few hundred cases that the doctors have given up on before they will utilize this theory. After all, that is the type of proof modern science demands.

My question is, why wait when none of the recommendations that come out of this theory can harm anyone? Why are we resistant to acknowledge that we really can have input into the evolution of our own potential cancer and the potential cancer of our loved ones. The input is not as simplistic as not eating hot dogs or not smoking. It is based upon a soul-searching frankness most people would prefer to avoid. And it is based upon taking the risk of possibly being rejected and hurt emotionally as things get rearranged.

Recent studies in England and America point out that cancer has a multistage development. The biologists are even now stating that the first stage might very well occur *early* in life. More and more the researchers are demonstrating molecular biological evidence of the instability of nucleic material as it relates to cancer. And those stubborn folk who refuse to get cancers while immersed in carcinogens and ignore anticancer nutrition remain an enigma to the research scientist.

Recently cancer is being blamed on a new culprit: survival, aging. We all know that the elderly in America are more prone to malignancies. But what of the ninety-year-old gentleman who sold us yogurt on TV and even had his mother come out of his home in the Crimea to confirm his claim that this dairy product was responsible for their longevity, as well as that of their neighbors. A friend of mine returned from fieldwork in the mountains of Peru to report that the Indians there frequently live to well past one hundred. As a matter of fact, one hundred is nothing unusual. This book has explained why in America the elderly are more vulnerable. It also has offered answers as to why in other societies survival is in itself not the cause of cancer.

The risk in pursuing a narrow frame of reference with regard to cancer is that you will wind up in blind alleys. While addressing the American Cancer Society's 25th Annual Science Writers' Seminar, noted cancer researcher and molecular biologist Dr. H. Rubin of the University of California at Berkeley pointed out that an obsessional "euphoria" with oncogenes (the minutia of the cell nucleus) will eventually prove to be another blind alley in this field. He has stated that a *new* medical biology will be needed to solve the mystery of cancer. I agree with this very respected scientist but would add that obsession with specifics such as oncogenes, nutrition, and carcinogens is an obstacle to integrating what is already known. This theory accomplishes that integration.

I believe that the ideas I have put forth can affect the disorder we call cancer. Their only side effect is cure.

Twenty years ago C. D. Darlington, addressing the First Oxford Chromosome Conference (1964), presented an adaptive hierarchy that also supports my theory. Basically, he stated that the physical hierarchy of molecule-gene-chromosome-organism-community corresponds to a living hierarchy. In my opinion, significant irritation at any point along this continuum will result in significant negative change. Thus, in acknowledging the instability of genetic material, we acknowledge molecular biology's contribution. But can we now see that *irritation* to the community can work its way down to the individual and then to the final point, the chemical nature of the genetic material?

I have one last suggestion for those of you who still doubt that cancer is a psychological and biological regression to infancy: visit your local hospital's oncology (cancer) unit and *see for yourself.* The most seriously regressed patients may be in diapers. They will have to be fed by others. Their physical coordination is close to nonexistent. Outbursts of upset or quiet withdrawal will mark their reaction to being overstimulated by irritants, usually provided by staff or relatives.

If all this fails to convince you, do one more thing: ask any of the physicians what characterizes the hormone levels of most tumors. They will say that they are elevated. Ask by how much. They will tell you that the *hormone levels are the same as in normally developing fetuses and newborns.*

So you see, I could not have waited.

Bibliography

Abse, D. W. et al., Personality and Behavioral Characteristics of Lung Cancer Patients. *J. Psychosom. Res.* 18, no. 2: (1974).

Abt, V. et al., The Impact of Mastectomy on Sexual Self-Image Attitudes and Behavior. *J. Sex. Ed. Ther.* 4: 43–47 (1978).

Ahlstroem, C. G., and Forsby, N. Sarcomas in Hamsters After Injection with Rous Chicken Tumor Material. *J. Exp. Med.* 115: 839–52 (1962).

Alexander, F., and French, T. M. *Psychoanalytic Therapy.* New York: Ronald, 1946.

Ames, B. Dietary Carcinogens and Anticarcinogens, *Science* 221: 1256–64 (1983).

Andrewes, C. H. The Work of the World Influenza Center. *J. of the Royal Ins. of Public Health* 15: 309–18 (1952).

———. Factors in Virus Evolution. *Adv. in Virus Res.* 4: 1–24 (1957).

———. The Complex Epidemiology of Respiratory Virus Infections. *Science* 146: 1274–77 (1964).

Appelbaum, S. Refusal to Take One's Own Medicine. *Bull. of the Menninger Clinic* 41, no. 6: 511–21 (Nov. 1977).

Bacon, C. L., Renniker, R., and Cutler, M. A Psychosomatic

Survey of Cancer of the Breast. *Psychosom. Med.* 14: 453–60 (1952).

Bartrop, R. W. et al., Depressed Lymphocyte Function after Bereavement. *Lancet* 1: 834–36 (1977).

Bellak, L. *Schizophrenia: A Review of the Syndrome.* New York: Grune & Stratton, 1958.

Berger, S. L. et al., Preparation of Interferon Messenger R.N.A. with the Use of Ribonucleic-vanadyl Complexes. *Methods Embryology* 79: 59–68 (1981).

Beringheli, F. Towards an Understanding of Cancer: Psychosomatic Phenomen. *Int. Mental Health Res. Newsletter* 16, no. 3: 3–6 (1947).

Bernstein, I., and Sigmundi, R. Tumor Anorexia: A Learned Food Aversion? *Science* 209 no. 4454: 416–18 (July 1980).

Bishop, J. M. The Molecular Biology of R.N.A. Tumor Viruses: A Physician's Guide. *N. Eng. J. of Med.* 303, no. 12: 675–82 (1980).

———. Enemies Within: The Genesis of Retrovirus Oncogenes. *Cell* 23, no. 1: 5–6 (1981).

———. Oncogenes. *Sci. Am.* 246, no. 3: (March 1982).

Bittner, J. J. Some Enigmas Associated with Genesis of Mammary Cancer in Mice. *Cancer Res.* 8: 625–39 (1948).

Boyd, W. The Spontaneous Regression of Cancer. *J. of Cancer Assoc. of Radiology* 8, 45, 62 (1957).

Buchland, F. E., and Tyrrell, D. A. J. Experiments on the Spread of Colds. *Laboratory Studies on the Dispersal of Nasal Secretions, J. Hygiene* 62: 365–77 (1965).

———. Experiments on the Spread of Colds. Studies in Volunteers with Coxsachic A 21. *J. Hygiene* 63: 327–43 (1965).

Buell, P., and Dunn, J. E. The Relative Impact of Smoking and Air Pollution on Lung Cancer. *Arch. Environ. Health* 15: 291 (1967).

Bulger, R. J. Doctors & Dying. *Arch. Intl. Med.* 112: 327–32 (1963).

Burkitt, D. A Sarcoma Involving the Jaws of African Children. *Brit. J. of Surgery* 46: 218–23 (1958).

Burnet, F. M., and Williams, S. W. Herpes Simplex: A New Point of View. *Med. J. of Australia 1: 637-42 (1939).*

Campbell, T. L. More Is Not Necessarily Better. *Natural Hist.* 90, no. 5: 12-26 (1981).

Cairns, J., Lyon J., and Skolnick M. Cancer Incidence in Defined Populations. *Banbury Report 4.* Cold Spring Harbor Laboratory (1980).

Cairns, J., and Palmer, S. Symposium on Food and Cancer. Columbia U. (1982).

Clemmsen, J., and Neilsen, A. Comparison of Age-adjusted Cancer Incidence Rates in Denmark and the United States. *J. Natl. Cancer Inst.* 19: 989 (1957).

Conference on Mind and Immunity, N.Y. Acad. of Med. (April 1982).

Cutler, E. Diet on Cancer. *Albany Med. Annals* (July-Aug., 1887).

Dattore, J. Premorbid Personality Characteristics Associated with Neoplasms: An Archival Approach. *Dissertation Abstr.* 41: (1981).

DeHaven, E., and Friend, C. Structure of Virus Particles Partially Purified from the Blood of Leukemic Mice. *Virology* 23: 119-24 (1964).

Donohue, V. Sexual Rehabilitation of Gynecologic Cancer Patients. *Med. Aspects of Human Sex* 51-52 (Feb. 1978).

Dowling, H. F. et al., Transmission of the Common Cold to Volunteers Under Controlled Conditions III The Effect of Chilling of the Subjects Upon Susceptibility. *Am. J. Hygiene* 37: 59-65 (1958).

Epstein, M. A., Achong, B. G., and Bars, Y. M. Virus Particles from Cultured Lymphocytes from Burkitts Lymphoma. *Lancet* 1: 702-3 (1964).

Epstein, S., and Swartz, J. Fallacies of Lifestyle Cancer Theories. *Nature* 289: no. 5794 (Jan. 1981).

Erving, J. *Neoplastic Disease: A Treatise on Tumors.* Phila. & London: W. B. Sanders, 1940.

Escalona, S. Emotional Development in the First Year of Life.

Problems of Infancy and Childhood, Conf. of Josiah Macy, Jr. Foundation. Ann Arbor, 1952.

Evans, E. *A Psychological Study of Cancer.* New York: Dodd Mead & Co., 1926.

Federn, P. *Ego Psychology and the Psychoses.* New York: Basic Books, 1952.

Federoff, N. V. *Controlling Elements in Maize, Mobile Genetic Elements.* Edited by J. Shapiro. Academic Press, 1983.

Federoff, N. V., Wessler, S., and Shure, S. Isolation of the Transposable Maize Controlling Elements Ac and Ds. *Cell* 35, no. 2: 235–42 (Nov. 1983).

Fenichel, O. *The Psychoanalytic Theory of Neurosis.* New York: W. W. Norton, 1945.

Fox, B. H. Premorbid Psychological Factors as Related to Cancer Incidence. *J. Behaviorial Med.* 1: 45–133 (1978).

Freud, S. *Repression* (1915), Standard Ed. 14: 141–58, London: Hogarth Press, 1957.

Friedman, M., and Rosenman, R. H. *Type A Behavior and Your Heart.* New York: Knopf, 1974.

Fuller, G. D. Current Status of Bio-Feedback in Clinical Practice. *Am. Psychologist* 39–48 (1978).

Galen. *De Tumoribus.* N.p., n.d.

Gates, C. A. *Manual for Cancer,* American Cancer Society (1978).

Gear, J. H. S. Coxsachic Virus Infections of the Newborn. *Progr. Med. Virology* 1: 106–21 (1958).

Gendron, D. *Enquiries into Nature, Knowledge, and Cure of Cancers.* London: 1701.

Gillihand, G. D. et al., Antibody-Disected Cytotoxic Agents: Use of Monoclonal Antibodies to Direct the Action of Toxin A Chains to Colorectal Carcinoma Cells. *Proc. Natl. Acad. of Sci.* U.S.A., 77, no. 8: 4539–43 (1980).

Giovacchini, P. Ego Equilibrium and Cancers of the Breast. In *Psychoanalysis of Character Disorders.* New York: Jason Aronson, 1975.

Green, E. Biofeedback and Voluntary Control of Internal States.

In *Frontiers of Science and Medicine,* edited by Henry Carlson. Chicago: Regency, 1975.

Green, R. G. On the Nature of Filterable Viruses. *Science* 82: 443-45 (1935).

Greene, W. Disease Response to Life Stress. *J. Amer. Med. Women's Assoc.* 20, no. 2: 133-40 (Feb. 1965).

———. Role of a Vicarious Object in the Adaptation to Object Loss. *Psychosom. Med.* 20, no. 5: 345-50, 1959.

———. The Psychosocial Setting of the Development of Leukemia and Lymphoma. *Annals of N.Y. Acad. of Sci.* 125: 794-801 (Jan. 21, 1966).

Greene, W., and Swisher, S. Psychological and Somatic Variables Associated with the Development and Course of Monozygotic Twins Discordant for Leukemia. *Annals of N.Y. Acad. of Sci.* 164, Article 2: 394-408 (Oct. 14, 1969).

Greenfield, L., et al., Nucleotide Sequence of the Structural Gene for Diphtheria Toxin Carried by Corynebacteriophage B. *Proc. Nat. Acad. of Sci.,* U.S.A. 80, no. 22: 6853-57 (Nov. 1983).

Greer, S., and Morris, T. Psychological Attributes of Women Who Develop Breast Cancer: A Controlled Study. *J. of Psychosom. Res.* 19: 147-53, 1975.

Grossarth-Matick, D. Psychosocial Predictors of Cancer and Internal Diseases: An Overview. *Psychotherapy and Psychosom.* 33, no. 3: 122-28 (1980).

———. Social Psychotherapy and Course of the Disease: First Experiences with Cancer Patients. *Psychotherapy and Psychosom.* 33, no. 3: 129-38 (1980).

Hanafusa, H. et al., The Defectiveness of the Rous Sarcoma Virus. *Proc. Natl. Acad. of Sci.* 49: 572-80 (1963).

Hemmes, J. H. et al., Virus Survival as a Seasonal Factor in Influenza and Poliomyelitis. *Nature* 188: 430-31 (1960).

Holden, C. Cancer and the Mind: How are They Connected. *Science* 200: 1363, 1978.

Holmes, T. H., and Madusa, M. Life Change and Illness Susceptibility Separation and Depression. *Am. Assoc. for Advancement of Sci.* 161–68 (1973).

Hope-Simpson, R. E. Discussion on the Common Cold. *Proc. Roy. Soc. Med.* 51: 267–72 (1958).

Horowitz, I. Enterline PE: Lung Cancer Among the Jews. *Am. J. Public Health* 60: 275–82 (1970).

Hughes, C. H. The Relations of Nervous Depression to the Development of Cancer. *St. Louis Medical and Surgical J.* May 1887.

Hull, R. N. et al., New Viral Agents Recovered from Monkey Tissue Culture Cells. *I Am. J. Hyg.* 65: 204–18.

Hunter, T., and Cooper J. A. Regulation of Cell Growth and Transformation by Tyrosive-specific Protein Kinases: The Search for Important Cellular Substrate Proteins. *Current Topics in Microbiology and Immunology.* 107: 125–61 (1983).

Issacs, A. Interferon. *Sci. Am.* 204: 51–57 (1961).

Issels, J. *Cancer: A Second Opinion.* London: Hadder & Stougleton, 1975.

Jackson, G., and Dowling H. Transmission of the Common Cold to Volunteers Under Controlled Conditions, IV Specific Immunity to the Common Cold. *J. of Clinical Investigation* 38: 762–69 (1959).

Jacobs, T., and Charles, E. Life Events and the Occurrence of Cancer in Children. *Psychosom. Med.* 42, no. 1: 11–24 (Jan. 1980).

Jacobson, E. *Depression: Comparative Studies of Normal, Neurotic, and Psychotic Conditions.* New York: International Universities Press, 1971.

Janerich, D. et al., Increased Leukemia, Lymphoma, and Spontaneous Abortion in Western New York Following a Flood Disaster. *Public Health Reports* 96: 350–56 (July-August 1981).

Johnson, A. et al., Lambda Repression and CRO-Component of an Efficient Molecular Switch. *Nature* 294, no. 5838: 217–23 (Nov. 1981).

Johnson, C. Cancer Incidence in an Area of Radioactive Fallout Downwind from the Nevada Test Site. *J. of Am. Med. Assoc.* 251, no. 2: 230–36 (Jan. 13, 1984).

Katz, J. et al., Psychoendocrine Considerations in Cancer of the Breast. *Annals of N.Y. Acad. of Sci.* 164: 509–16 (1969).

Kaye, J., Appel, M., and Joseph, R. Attitudes of Medical Students and Residents Toward Cancer. *J. of Psych.* 107, no. 1: 87–96 (1981).

Keller, A. Cellular Types, Survival, Race Nativity, Occupations, Habits, and Associated Diseases in the Pathogenesis of Lip Cancer. *Am. J. Epidemiol.* 91: 486–99 (1970).

Kernberg, O. *Borderline Conditions and Pathological Narcissism.* New York: Jason Aronson, 1975.

Kerr, M. Emotional Factors in Physical Illness: A Multigenerational Prospective. *Family* 7: 59–66 (1980).

King, H., Diamond E., Bailar, and J. C. III. Cancer Mortality and Religious Preference. *Milbank Mem. Fund Q.* 43: 349–58 (1965).

Kissen, D. M., and Eysenck, H. G. Personality in Male Lung Cancer Patients *J. Psychosom. Res.* 6: 123 (1962).

Kissen, D. M., and Rao, L. Steroid Excretion Patterns and Personality in Lung Cancer. *Annals of N.Y. Acad. of Sci.* 164: 476–82 (1969).

Klopfer, B. Psychological Variables in Human Cancer. *J. Projective Techniques* 21: 331–40 (1957).

Koocher, G. et al., Psychological Adjustment Among Pediatric Cancer Survivors. *J. Child Psych. and Psychiatry and Allied Disciplines* 21, no. 2: 163–73 (April 1980).

Kubler-Ross, E. *On Death and Dying.* New York: MacMillian Co., 1969.

Laidlow, P. P. *Virus Diseases and Viruses.* Cambridge: Cambridge U. Press, 1938.

Lasagna, L. The Doctor and the Dying Patient. *J. Chron. Dis.* 22, no. 1069: 65–68.

Leboyer. *Birth Without Violence.* New York: Knopf, 1975.

LeShan, L. Psychological States as Factors in Development of Malignant Disease: A Critical Review. *J. Nat. Cancer Inst.* 22: 1-18 (1959).

_____. An Emotional Life History Pattern Associated with Neoplastic Disease. *Annals of N.Y. Aca. of Sci.* 125: 780-93 (1966).

_____. *You Can Fight for Your Life.* New York: M. Evans, 1977.

Lidwell, O., and Williams, R. The Epidemiology of the Common Cold. *J. of Hygiene* 59: 309-34 (1961).

Lyon, J., et al., Low Cancer Incidence and Mortality in Utah. *Cancer* 39: 2608-18 (1977).

_____. Cancer Incidence in Mormons and Non-Mormons in Utah, 1966-1970. *N. Eng. J. Med.* 294: 129-33 (1976).

_____. Cancer Incidence in Mormons and Non-Mormons in Utah during 1967-1975. *J. Natl. Cancer Inst.* 65: 1055-61 (1980).

Mackintosh, S. Incidence of Breast and Cervical Cancer Among Women and Selected Social and Psychological Variables. *Dissertation Abstr.* 40: (1980).

MacMahon, B. et al., Ethnic Differences in the Incidence of Leukemia. *Blood* 12: 1-10 (1957).

_____. Age at First Birth and Breast Cancer Risk. *Bull. WHO* 43: 209-21 (1970).

_____. Coffee and Cancer of the Pancreas. *N. Engl. J. Med.* 304: 630-33 (1981).

Mahler, M. On Child Psychosis and Schizophrenia. *Psychoanalytic Study of the Child* 7: 286-305 (1952).

Mahler, M., and Elkisch, P. Some Observations on Disturbances of the Ego in a Case of Infantile Psychosis. *Psychoanalytic Study of the Child* 8: 252-61 (1953).

Mahler, M. et al. *The Psychological Birth of the Human Infant.* New York: Basic Books, 1975.

Margolis, B. Narcissistic Countertransference: Emotional Availability and Case Management. *J. Modern Psychoanalysis* 3, no. 2: (1978).

Mason, J. W. Psychologic Stress and Endocrine Function. In *Topics in Psychoendocrinology,* edited by E. J. Sachar. New York: Grune & Stratton, 1965.

Mason, T. H., and McKay, F. W. *U.S. Cancer Mortality by County: 1950-1969* DHEW publication no. (NIH) 74-615, Washington, DC: USGPO, 1974.

Masson, P. *Human Tumors,* Detroit: Wayne State University Press, 1970.

McClintock, B. Mutable Loci in Maize. *Carnegie Inst. of Wash. Yearbook.* 47: 159 (1948).

————. Mutable Loci in Maize. *Carnegie Inst. of Wash. Yearbook.* 48: 142-43 (1949).

————. Chromosome Organization and Genetic Expression. Cold Spring Harbor Symposium on Quantitative Biology. 16: 40 (1951).

————. Induction of Instability of Selected Loci in Maize. *Genetics.* 38: 579-99 (1953).

————. The Control of Gene Action in Maize. Brookhaven Symposium in Biology. 18: 162-84 (1965).

————. Modified Gene Expressions Induced by Transposable Elements. In *Mobilization and Reassembly of Genetic Information,* edited by W. Scott. et al. New York: Academic Press, 1980.

Meares, A. Vivid Visualization and Dim Visual Awareness in the Regression of Cancer in Meditation. *J. Am. Soc. of Psychosom. Dentistry and Med.* 25, no. 3: 85-99 (1978).

Mider, G. Some Aspects of Nitrogen and Energy Metabolism in Cancer Subjects: A Review. *Cancer Res.* 11: 821-29 (1951).

Milann, D., and Smithie, W. A Bacteriological Study of Colds on an Isolated Tropical Island. *J. Exp. Med.* 53: 733-52 (1931).

Mitchell, S. Twilight of the Gods. *Contemporary Psychoanalysis* 15, no. 1: 170-89 (1979).

Morrison, S. Partition of Energy Expenditure Between Host and Tumors. *Cancer Res.* 31: 98-107 (1971).

————. Limited Capacity for Motor Activity as a Cause for Declining Food Intake in Cancer. *J. Nat. Cancer Inst.* 51: 1535-39 (1973).

———. Control of Food Intake in Cancer Cathexis: A Challenge and a Tool. *Physiology and Behavior* 17: 705–14 (1976).

Nagera, H. *Basic Psychoanalytic Concepts on the Libido Theory.* et al. New York: Basic Books, 1969.

Nakara, W. A Chemical Basis for Tumor Host Relations. *J. Nat. Cancer Inst.* 24: 77–86 (1960).

National Office of Vital Statistics. Mortality from Selected Causes by Marital Status, U.S. 1949–1951. *Vital Health Stat.* 39: 301–429 (1956).

Nevers, P., and Saidler, H. Transposable Genetic Elements as Agents of Gene Instability and Chromosomal Rearrangements. *Nature* 268: 109 (1977).

Newell, V. Distribution of Cancer Mortality Among Ethnic Subgroups of the White Population of New York City, 1953-1958. *J. Natl. Cancer Inst.* 26: 405–17 (1961).

Nunberg, H. *Principles of Psychoanalysis.* New York: International U. Press, 1955.

Pabo, C., and Lewis, M. The Operator-Binding Domain of Lambda Repression: Structure and DNA Recognition. *Nature* 298, no. 5873: 443–47 (July 1982).

Parens, H. An Explanation of the Relations of Instinctual Drives and the Symbiosis/Separation-Individuation Process. *J. Am. Psychoan. Assoc.* 28, no. 1: (1980).

Parker, C. The First Year of Bereavement: A Longitudinal Study of the Reaction of London Widows to the Death of their Husbands. *Psychiatry* 33: 444–67 (1970).

———. Comment: Communication and Cancer: A Social Psychiatrist's View. *Soc. Sci. and Med.* 8, no. 4: 189–90 (1974).

Patel, M. et al., Psychological Manifestation in Cancer Patients, Preliminary Study. *Indian J. Clin. Psych.* 7, no. 2: 147–50 (Sept. 1980).

Paul, J., and Freese, H. Epidemiological Bactriological Study of Common Colds in Isolated Arctic Community. *Am. J. Hygiene* 17: 517–35 (1933).

Pepper, C. *We the Victors.* New York: Doubleday, 1984.

Ptashne, M. et al., How the Lambda Repression and CRO Work. *Cell* 19, no. 1: 1–11 (Jan. 1980).

————. Lambda Repression and CRO-Components of an Efficient Molecular Switch. *Nature* 294, no. 5838: 217–23 (Nov. 1981).

Ptashne, M., Johnson A., and Pabo C. A Genetic Switch in a Bacterial Virus. *Sci. Am.* 247, no. 5: 128–40 (Nov. 1982).

Ramos-Alvarez, M., and Rubin, A. Intestinal Viral Flora of Healthy Children Demonstrated by Monkey Kidney Tissue Culture. *Am. J. Public Health* 46: 295–99 (1956).

Riley, V. Mouse Mammary Tumors: Attraction of Incidence as Apparent Function of Stress. *Science* 189: 465–67 (Aug. 1975).

Rogers, S. and Rous P. Joint Action of a Chemical Carcinogen and a Neoplastic Virus to Induce Cancer in Rabbits. *J. Mp. Med.* 93: 459–85 (1951).

Rosch, P. Mind and Cancer. *Lancet* 1: 130–32 (1979).

————. Stress and Cancer: Disease of Adaptation. In *Cancer, Stress and Death,* edited by Tache et al. 187–212, New York, 1979.

Sabini, et al., An Inner View of Illness: The Dreams of Two Cancer Patients. *J. Analytical Psych.* 26, no. 2: 123–50 (1981).

Schleifer, S. et al. Suppression of Lymphocyte Stimulation Following Bereavement. *J. Am. Med. Assoc.* 250, no. 3: 374–77 (July 1983).

Schmale, A., and Iker, H. The Psychological Setting of Uterine Cervical Cancer. *Annals of N.Y. Acad. of Sci.* 125: 807–15 (1966).

Selnizer, S. Stress Can Be Good for You. *New York Magazine,* Aug. 1982.

Seyli, H. *The Stress of Life.* New York: McGraw-Hill, 1956.

Shapot, V. Some Biochemical Aspects of the Relationship Between the Host. *Adv. Cancer Res.* 15: 253–86 (1972).

Shope, R. A Transmissible Tumor-like Condition in Rabbits. *J. Exp. Med.* 56: 793–802 (1932).

Simonton, B., Simonton S., and Creighton J. *Getting Well Again.* Los Angeles: J. P. Tacher, 1978.

Sklar, L., and Anisman, H. Social Stress Influences Tumor Growth. *Psychosom. Med.* 42, no. 3: 347–65 (May 1980).

————. Stress and Cancer. *Psychological Bull.* 89, no. 3: 369–406 (May 1981).

Smith, W., Andrewes, C., and Laidlow, P. A Virus Obtained from Influenza Patients. *Lancet* 2, 66–68 (1933).

Snow, H. *The Reappearance of Cancer after Apparent Extirpation.* London: J. & A. Churchill, 1870.

Solomon, G. Emotions, Stress, the Central Nervous System, and Immunity. *Annals of N.Y. Acad. of Sci.* 164, no. 2: 335–43 (1969).

Spence, D. Lawfulness in Lexical Choice: A Natural Experiment. *J. Am. Psychoan. Assoc.* 28, no. 1: 115–32 (1980).

Spicer, J., and Gustavus S. Mormon Fertility Through Half a Century: Another Test of the Americanization Hypothesis. *Soc. Biol.* 21: 70 (1974).

Spiegel, D., Bloom, J., and Yalom, I. Group Support for Patients with Metastic Cancer: A Randomized Prospective Outcome Study. *Arch. of Gen. Psychiatry* 48, no. 5: 527–33 (1981).

Spitz, R. Hospitalism: A Followup Report. *Psychoanalytic Study of The Child* 2: 113–17 (1945).

————. Hospitalism: An Inquiry into the Genesis of Psychiatric Conditions in Early Childhood. *Psychoanalytic Study of the Child.* 53–74 (1945).

————. Anaclitic Depression. *Psychoanalytic Study of the Child* 2: 313–42 (1946).

————. *The First Year of Life.* New York: International U. Press, 1965.

Spotnitz, H. *Modern Psychoanalysis of the Schizophrenic Patient.* New York: Grune & Stratton, 1969.

————. Psychotherapy of Preoedipal Conditions. New York: Jason Aronson, 1976.

Stefansson, V. *Cancer: A Disease of Civilization.* New York: Hill & Wang, 1960.

Stone, L. *The Psychoanalytic Situation.* New York: International U. Press, 1961.

Sugano, H., and Sasano, N. (Chairpeople). Symposia on Cancer and Hormones, Proceedings of the Japanese Cancer Association, 39th Annual Meeting, G.A.M.M.—*Jap. J. of Cancer Res.*, Tokyo, 1980.

Terris, M., and Oalmann, M. Carcinoma of the Cervix: An Epidemiologic Study. *JAMA* 174: 1847-51 (1960).

Terris, M., Wilson, F. et al., Epidemiology of Cancer of the Cervix V. The Relationship of Coitus to Carcinoma of the Cervix. *Am. J. Public Health* 57: 840-47 (1967).

Theologides, A. Pathogenesis of Cachexia in Cancer: A Review and Hypothesis. *Cancer* 29: 484-88 (1972).

Thomas, C., and Greenstreet, R. Psychological Characteristics in Youth as Predictors of Five Disease States: Suicide, Mental Illness, Hypertension, Coronary Heart Disease, and Tumors. *Johns Hopkins Med. J.* 132: 16-43 (1973).

Thomas, L. Cellular and Hormonal Aspects of the Hypersensitive States. In Symposia of the Section in Microbiology, edited by H. S. Lawrence, N.Y. Academy of Med., Casoil, London, 1959.

Tresillian Fire, M. *Does Diet Cure Cancer?* Northampshire: Thorsons, Willingborough, 1976.

Tyrrell, D., and Bynoc, M. Some Further Virus Isolations from Common Colds. *Brit. Med. J.* 1: 393-97 (1961).

Vachon, M., and Llyadd, W. Applying Psychiatric Techniques to

Patients with Cancer. *Hosp. and Comm. Psychiatry* 28, no. 8: 582–84 (1976).

Wartin, A. Heredity With Reference to Carcinoma. *Arch. Intl. Med.* 12: 546–55 (1913).

Watson, C., and Schuld, D. Psychosomatic Factors in the Etiology of Neoplasms. *J. Cons. and Clin. Psych.* 43, no. 3: 455–61 (1977).

Weinberg, R. The Secrets of Cancer Cells. *Atlantic* 252, no. 2: (August 1983).

Weinstock, C. Recent Progress in Cancer Psychobiology and Psychiatry. *J. Am. Soc. Psychosom. Dent. and Med.* 24, no, 1: 4–14 (1977).

Winder, P. *Minimal Brain Dysfunction in Children.* Nev ⸢ York: Wily-Interscience, 1971.

Winnicott, D. *Primary Maternal Preoccupation, Collected Papers,* New York: Basic Books, 300–305 (1958).

Wise, T. N. Sexual Functioning in Neoplastic Disease. *Med. Aspects of Human Sexuality.* 16–31 (March 1978).

Young, J. L. et al., Cancer Incidence and Mortality in the United States. 1973-1976. DHEW pub no. (NIH) 78-1837, NCI, 1978, Bethesda, Maryland.

Young, V., and Newberne, P. Vitamins and Cancer Prevention: Issues and Dilemmas. *Cancer* 47: 1226–40 (1981).

This is only a sampling of the relevant literature on this topic. To include all references would require a listing of 500 to 1,000 articles and books.

In addition to what is listed, I would like to mention the innumerable phone conversations with physicians, research biologists, nutritionists, and psychoanalysts. I tapped into the libraries and minds of many hospitals throughout the country. Particular thanks is extended to the oncologists, neuropathologists, pediatricians, and neonatologists who took time from their overwhelming schedules to answer my technical questions.

Index

Index